KV-240-319

amelia lawson   james lawson

breast cancer

can you prevent it?

McGRAW-HILL BOOK COMPANY Sydney
New York San Francisco Auckland Bogotá
Caracas Lisbon London Madrid Mexico City
Milan Montreal New Delhi San Juan
Singapore Tokyo Toronto

McGraw·Hill Australia

A Division of The McGraw·Hill Companies

Medicine is an ever-changing science. As new research and clinical experience broaden our knowledge, changes in treatment and drug therapy are required. The editors and the publisher of this work have checked with sources believed to be reliable in their efforts to provide information that is complete and generally in accord with the standards accepted at the time of publication. However, in view of the possibility of human error or changes in medical sciences, neither the editors, nor the publisher, nor any other party who has been involved in the preparation or publication of this work warrants that the information contained herein is in every respect accurate or complete. Readers are encouraged to confirm the information contained herein with other sources.

Text © 1999 James Lawson and Amelia Lawson
Illustrations and design © 1999 McGraw-Hill Book Company Australia Pty Limited
Additional owners of copyright are named in on-page credits.

Apart from any fair dealing for the purposes of study, research, criticism or review, as permitted under the *Copyright Act*, no part may be reproduced by any process without written permission. Enquiries should be made to the publisher, marked for the attention of the Permissions Editor, at the address below.

Every effort has been made to trace and acknowledge copyright material. Should any infringement have occurred accidentally the authors and publishers tender their apologies.

Copying for educational purposes
Under the copying provisions of the *Copyright Act*, copies of parts of this book may be made by an educational institution. An agreement exists between the Copyright Agency Limited (CAL) and the relevant educational authority (Department of Education, university, TAFE, etc.) to pay a licence fee for such copying. It is not necessary to keep records of copying except where the relevant educational authority has undertaken to do so by arrangement with the Copyright Agency Limited.

For further information on the CAL licence agreements with educational institutions, contact the Copyright Agency Limited, Level 19, 157 Liverpool Street, Sydney NSW 2000. Where no such agreement exists, the copyright owner is entitled to claim payment in respect of any copies made.

Enquiries concerning copyright in McGraw-Hill publications should be directed to the Permissions Editor at the address below.

National Library of Australia Cataloguing-in-Publication data:

Lawson, James S.
    Breast cancer: can you prevent it?

    Bibliography
    ISBN 0 07 470723 X.

    1. Breast–Cancer–Prevention. 2. Breast–Cancer. I. Lawson, Amelia J., 1972- .II. Title.l

616.99449052

Published in Australia by
McGraw-Hill Book Company Australia Pty Limited
4 Barcoo Street, Roseville NSW 2069, Australia
Acquisitions Editor: Kristen Baragwanath
Production Editors: Sybil Kesteven, Jo Rudd
Designer: Jenny Pace Design
Cover design: Jenny Pace Design
Illustrator: Alan Laver, Shelly Communication
Typeset by Jenny Pace Design
Printed by Star Printery, Australia

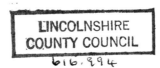

LINCOLNSHIRE
COUNTY COUNCIL

616.994

foreword

❧

P rofessor James Lawson is a distinguished academic and a talented writer. He has an unusual ability to internalise a vast amount of information and identify what is likely to be important among the many reported research results. Although we have never met, we share many ideas about the causes of breast cancer and the possibilities for prevention. I have also never had the privilege to meet his daughter, Amelia Lawson, but her intellectual grace and sensitivity are reflected in her writing. For these reasons, I did not hesitate to write a foreword to their book on the possibilities for prevention of breast cancer. My willingness, however, turned into enthusiasm after I had the opportunity to read an early draft of their book.

The book was written for women and the men who love them. It requires no biomedical background and avoids scientific jargon. Nevertheless, it is a genuinely scientific piece of work that could be extremely useful not only for the educated layperson but also for the qualified professional. The authors attribute the ideas presented in their work to many investigators, including myself, but the synthesis is distinctly their own—and an elegant synthesis it is. They present the evidence concerning the aetiology and preventability of breast cancer in a coherent authoritative way, but at the same time they write a fascinating chronicle of the gigantic research effort by many thousands of investigators who have dedicated their professional lives to the understanding of the causes of breast cancer. The book starts in a dramatic way but it is essentially optimistic—there are already actions that can be taken to reduce the risk for breast cancer and there are many highly promising leads for an eventual elucidation of the breast cancer enigma.

This is a valuable book that may change the lives of many women and the perspectives of many investigators. I strongly recommend it for specialists and non-specialists, professionals and non-professionals, and for both women and the men who love them.

Boston, August 1998

Dimitrios Trichopoulos, MD
Vincent L Gregory Professor of Cancer Prevention and
    Professor of Epidemiology
Harvard School of Public Health, Boston, MA, USA

the authors

James S. Lawson

James Lawson is a 64 year old professor who teaches public health and management to graduate students at the University of New South Wales in Sydney, Australia. Although he began professional life as a paediatrician, he has spent most of his career as a senior public health and hospital manager. He has been a pioneer in the use of epidemiology as the basis for health service planning and the redirection of resources into health promotion activities. Much of this work has been published in the scientific literature and in his many books.

He has worked in developing countries for many years, initially as a member of the Red Cross medical relief teams in the Congo in 1961, followed by a year as a paediatrician in Papua New Guinea in 1964. During the past 15 years he has worked as a World Health Organisation (WHO) consultant in many countries. It was this experience that drew his attention to breast cancer because of the dramatic differences in the incidence of breast cancer in the countries he worked in. He observed at first hand that Japan, China, Hong Kong and the Philippines had very low incidences of breast cancer compared with Australia, Canada, the US, the UK and other Western countries. When preparing policy papers for the WHO he found that these observations, while well known in epidemiologic

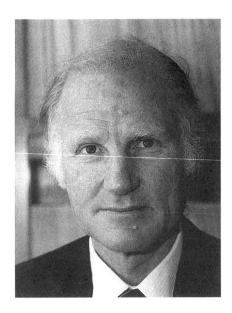

circles, were not known by senior health policy makers and certainly not by the general public.

He also found that there was little interest in the prevention of breast cancer and that virtually all available resources were being directed to early detection and treatment. Such an approach has achieved modest progress in the fight against breast cancer but, in the absence of any strategies for prevention, the problem remains a formidable one. Hence this book, which he has written with his daughter, Amelia. The book aims to review the facts and to offer some practical action that can be taken to begin the long process of preventing breast cancer.

This is the fourth book by James Lawson published by McGraw-Hill. His previous, highly successful books with McGraw-Hill are: *Public Health Australia*, 1991; *Health Promotion Strategies*, co-authored by Garry Egger and Ross Spark in 1992; and *From Clinician to Manager*, co-authored by Arie Rotem and Philip Bates in 1996. In 1969 he wrote the first Australian book advocating health system reform.

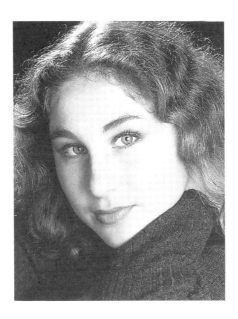

Amelia J. Lawson

Amelia is a 26 year old graduate, also of the University of New South Wales. She trained as a teacher of English and Drama and has spent the past three years teaching the English to write and speak English in London. She is currently working in the film and television industry in Sydney. She does not claim to have special knowledge about breast cancer. Her role in the creation of this book has been to provide a woman's perspective and, of course, to improve her father's writing skills.

While both father and daughter have collaborated throughout the writing of this book, it will be obvious that some of the personal experiences are those of Amelia.

contents

modern women and breast cancer

How many women are affected by breast cancer each year? How many more people are affected by and through those women? Most of us know someone, or know of someone, who has developed breast cancer—but how many of us know exactly what that means or have a clue as to why it happened at all?

If you picked up any Cancer Council booklet from your local health clinic you would be offered 52 pages of information titled *Understanding Breast Cancer*. If you looked a little further you would discover that the booklet 'answers the questions most people ask and gives practical tips on how to cope with your treatment and feelings'. This is undeniably pertinent and valuable information for women and their families. But what about the section that tells you what you can do to prevent breast cancer? Enquire a little further and you will discover that there is currently no accepted policy for the prevention of breast cancer in any country in the world. In place of such a policy, communities have been educated to rely on 'early detection' methods, such as mammography and self-examination, to protect themselves. Why is this the case? We have long accepted the adage 'prevention is better than cure' and, with the advanced state of medical knowledge, have been able to apply it. We know that not smoking will help prevent lung cancer and we know that exercise and a low-fat diet will help prevent heart disease. But what about breast cancer?

More than 38 500 scientific papers concerning breast cancer were published during the last decade alone. These included studies into the patterns of breast cancer in relation to the food we eat, age at first period, when we reproduce, when we go through menopause, our socioeconomic status, our weight, our height, whether we smoke and what country we live in. Despite this huge investment of time, money and ability we seem to be no closer to developing an offensive against one of the biggest killers of women in the Western world. Or are we?

Because, at this stage, current knowledge about the possible causes of breast cancer, and the follow-up investigations into prevention, are almost wholly confined to a small group of public health scientists whose work's progress is published in obscure journals, it is very difficult for doctors and health care workers to gain a comprehensive overview of the breast cancer situation.

When even the experts are uncertain and ill-informed the reality is that those outside the medical arena are even less likely to know the breast cancer facts. Yes, the common person has access to public health information pamphlets, and when you find them insufficiently informative, yes, more detailed information is out there—if you are interested enough to dedicate yourself to two years' research. A difficult situation, but one not without a solution.

This book is unique for several reasons. The most important of these is that it offers women the first comprehensive listing and discussion of preventive measures against breast cancer. These are not 'quick fix' solutions, and there remains to be found a breast cancer antidote, but they provide women with the opportunity to take some control of their body's fight against possible breast cancer.

A plan of disease prevention is based largely on determining the cause of the disease. In the case of breast cancer, many possible causes have been considered. Research studies have investigated whether there is a relationship between breast cancer development and these possible causes, and what this relationship might be.

Using this book as a guide, women are given the opportunity to protect themselves and also offered the information that will allow them to determine their current level of breast cancer risk. The book considers each factor that is thought to influence the development of breast cancer. In order to dispel certain breast cancer myths, and to give the reader an understanding of the facts, we summarise the theories behind the investigations and give a synopsis of the results. Studies show that some of the factors have no relationship to breast cancer at all, whereas others have been found to carry some influence. By providing a 'risk factor' for each of these factors (e.g. women who have late onset of menopause have a 15% higher chance of developing breast cancer than women who go through menopause early), women can evaluate themselves in relation to each factor and determine their own level of risk.

Every attempt has been made to offer this information at a 'user-friendly' level. The aim is to provide readers with the tools of comprehension. To achieve this, the book attempts to address all areas of the breast cancer issue, from the basic to the complicated, with equal weight and clarity.

Using plain English, we give information on how the breast is constructed, and introduce the reader to the process of breast cancer development and treatment. We define, and place in context, terms relevant to the topic—terms you may be familiar with, without being certain of their meaning. Many of the facts and issues are repeated in various sections of the book to ease the burden on your recall of the more complex matters.

Understanding the make-up of our own bodies and knowing the relevant language is the first step towards untangling the breast cancer facts from the fictions. You will be given the opportunity to learn about the health scientists whose lives have been devoted to researching breast cancer, the theories they have developed and investigated over the last century, the weaknesses and strengths of these investigations and the possible discoveries that will be made in the future. You will be one of the first to learn about the latest development, one that pinpoints a previously unknown relationship between breast cancer and babies. Most importantly, you will be given the opportunity to decide for yourself, based on the information provided, what you need to know about breast cancer and how best you can use that knowledge to protect yourself and your family.

We begin with the story of Elizabeth Sutherland. This is not her real name, and some of the details of her story have been altered to preserve her family's privacy, but she was a real person. Her story is typical of women of our time who have contracted and died from breast cancer. Her experience and her tragedy offer many clues to the cause and control of breast cancer.

elizabeth
sutherland

Dunolly, a rural town in Victoria, Australia, is not much of a place these days. If you consult a travel book, Dunolly generally merits little more than a couple of lines and even then the credit is by association. The 'Welcome Stranger', the largest nugget of gold ever discovered in the world (136 pounds, so big it had to be cut up to fit on the scales) was found in Moliagul, a town a short way from Dunolly, in 1869.

More gold was found in this area than anywhere else in Australia. During its heyday there were some 30 000 prospectors in the area, each one desperately digging and panning and dreaming he would be the next to make his fortune. With the gold-mad diggers came their families. This meant big business to a small country town and life in Dunolly flourished. General stores sprang up, stocking everything you could possibly need, two new hotels opened, the main street was repaved and the local school's enrolment trebled (two new schoolrooms had to be erected to cater for all the extra pupils).

Dunolly's prosperity was short-lived, however. No more great discoveries were made and the fortune hunters vanished as quickly as they had appeared. By the 1940s Dunolly was once more a quiet rural town, a suitably isolated place for a dedicated Methodist minister to find his calling. Such a minister was the fine and upstanding Reverend Sutherland, supported by his equally upstanding young wife. The couple came to Dunolly so that Reverend Sutherland could take on the position of minister to Dunolly's large Methodist congregation.

It was almost two years after their arrival that the Sutherlands' first child was born—a 9 pound 3 ounce daughter. The proud parents decided to name the golden-haired little girl Elizabeth, after the elder of the little English princesses they had read so much about. Although life in Australia was very different from the world they had known in England, the Sutherlands were young, healthy and dedicated to their god-given mission. Of necessity they quickly became accustomed to the differences of their new surrounds, and the small family settled with remarkably little fuss and bother.

The impression most of us have of smallish rural towns like Dunolly is that they are just that—small-town, a little small-minded and very behind the times. Yet the young, and increasingly pregnant, Mrs Sutherland bought and read all the new baby books that she heard were the rage with forward-thinking young mothers in Sydney and Melbourne, including 'America's paediatrician', Dr Spock's *Baby and Child Care*.

The subsequently well informed Mrs Sutherland was mindful of taking regular exercise and careful with the food she ate. In those days this meant she went for an hour-long walk every day, ate red meat twice a day, and consumed plenty of whole milk and cheese 'for the baby's bones', plus apples and stewed rhubarb for afters.

Despite all this modern-day knowledge and care, Mrs Sutherland's birth was a painfully difficult one. The contractions began late on Sunday evening, a week before the baby was due, and continued intermittently for nearly 12 hours. Severe contractions over the next six hours brought the first real progress and finally, at approximately 4 o'clock in the afternoon, Elizabeth Esther, a rather large first baby, was born into the midwife's arms at the local district hospital.

Mrs Sutherland was understandably exhausted. She had suffered a vaginal tear and, because of shortages due to the war, had to have stitches without anaesthetic. However, at the age of 25 she was physically fit and healthy enough to make a thorough and joyously rapid recovery.

Mother and daughter quickly settled into a regular routine. The little girl was breastfed every three hours (almost to the minute) according to the hospital policy of doing it the 'Truby-King' way. Truby King was a male New Zealand baby doctor, quite as unable to give birth as Dr Spock was. Like Dr Spock, however, he had watched enough gestations, procreations and complications to feel he had a pretty good idea how best to do it. His two books, charmingly dogmatic and didactic as they were, recommended the rapid introduction of solids at the age of four months. When Elizabeth did not put on the weight required by the books, she was given bottled cow's milk as 'supplements'.

All this food achieved the correct result—Elizabeth grew rapidly. In those days the baby growth charts were based on the way British babies had grown during the 1920s and 1930s. Within six months, Elizabeth had grown faster than nearly all her British counterparts and continued to do so for many years.

Australia had an agricultural economy and even during the darkest days of the war, with only the American fleet standing in the way of a Japanese invasion, the Sutherlands continued to eat well. The only food they missed were special treats such as icecream and sugared cherries, but Mrs Sutherland was a capable woman and she made her own treats, usually custard and cream, with a curl of red apple peel on top.

Elizabeth was a lovely child. She looked like neither parent, but seemed to have a little bit of both in her finely featured face. Unlike her reserved and introverted parents she was a 'smiley' little girl who would initiate conversation with anyone—and usually have them laughing in minutes, much to the bemusement of her embarrassed mother.

Elizabeth grew quickly. By the age of 11 she was as tall as her mother and at 12 she began her first menstrual cycle. Although she joined in sports as part of her school's curriculum, she was not very good at any of them and found she did not enjoy any of the competitive games. Instead, Elizabeth became a great reader. She consumed the works of Jane Austen, Henry James and the Brontës and, if she had been forced to choose her favourite, the great romantic in her would have picked *Wuthering Heights*.

When she was 14 Elizabeth discovered another great passion. She realised that you did not need to be particularly good at sports to enjoy them. Boys played sports (well, the best ones did, anyway) and, although they generally did not fulfil all her romantic expectations, Elizabeth spent the next few years happily falling in and out of love from the sidelines. She was a confident girl and did not seem surprised that most of the boys she admired so much seemed to reciprocate her admiration.

Had Elizabeth grown up in a big city like Sydney or Melbourne, where the introduction of the contraceptive pill was resulting in greater sexual liberation and greater freedom for women, her future may have been altogether different. But things were a little slower in Dunolly and, as a young middle-class girl, Elizabeth's experience of being in love was limited to feeling emotional and romantic. And so, despite her popularity and the many Friday night opportunities, Elizabeth remained relatively sexually inexperienced until the evening of her marriage in 1968 at the age of twenty-one.

Elizabeth had met her future husband while working as a scientist in a Melbourne hospital laboratory. John Wright—Jack to his friends—was a medical pathologist, tall, quite good looking and suitably ambitious. Friends often said that the couple 'complemented' one another perfectly and it came as no surprise to anyone when they announced their engagement.

Elizabeth felt she had outgrown Dunolly and so decided to hold the wedding in Melbourne, much to her mother's disappointment. The special day took Elizabeth and Mrs Sutherland six months to plan and when it finally took place, at the local Uniting Church in South Yarra (by 1968 Australian Methodists and Presbyterians had joined to become the Uniting Church), the eighty guests, three bridesmaids, two groomsmen, one best man and a flower girl, plus, of course, the bride and groom, all arrived and performed to perfection.

Even though she was still only 21, nearly 22, Elizabeth could not wait to have a baby. Getting pregnant was no problem and within ten months of the wedding her first son was born. Elizabeth loved being at home with the baby and was a natural mother. Her only real difficulty was breastfeeding. She found that her nipples quickly became sore and dry and would sometimes crack. The baby was often irritable as a result and both Elizabeth and John got very little sleep. Like her mother, who had also had breastfeeding problems, Elizabeth resorted to a baby bottle. This quickly solved the nipple problem, and the sleep problem, and both mother and son put on weight.

Elizabeth became a city girl, living in Hawthorn, one of the leafier Melbourne suburbs. She spent her days looking after her baby, organising the household and being a wife to her new husband. It was all very normal and traditional for a successful Australian family of the 1960s. They spent most evenings at home. Elizabeth had been given a Margaret Fulton cookbook as a wedding present and was discovering, with some trial and error, the satisfaction of preparing a meal for her very own family. Her mother had rarely let her into the kitchen of the family home and so Elizabeth was a culinary novice. She quickly learnt the beautiful simplicity of a roast dinner and it was not uncommon for the Wright family to enjoy a variation on the roast theme three times a week. Roast chicken, roast lamb or roast beef, roasted (and occasionally boiled) vegetables followed by stewed fruit and custard. Not exactly *haute cuisine* but more than adequate for the family of three.

The passing years brought an improvement in Elizabeth's cooking and an enlargement in her family. By 1979 there were three Wright children, two boys and one girl, all growing rapidly and healthily. Elizabeth and her husband decided to try for one more girl and in 1981 they were blessed with the birth of Anastasia Rose. By this stage Elizabeth was quite expert in the nurturing of babies. She no longer read any baby books but cared for her children as her instincts and experience told her.

Breastfeeding was no longer difficult but Elizabeth began to suffer some discomfort in her left breast which worried her. After a quick examination, the doctor in the local clinic prescribed antibiotics. He could feel a slight thickening of the breast tissue and made the sensible judgment that Elizabeth had an infection.

The pain eased and Elizabeth continued to breastfeed the new baby. She could still feel the thickness in the breast tissue and sometimes thought that maybe it was slightly bigger than before. The doctor had not seemed unduly worried so Elizabeth decided it was nothing and hoped it would go away when she stopped breastfeeding.

When the dull ache returned, fear overcame denial. Elizabeth returned to the clinic where, after a second examination, the doctor recommended a **biopsy**. He explained that a biopsy involved the removal of a piece of the lump with a specially designed cutting needle. The sample was then analysed under a microscope by the pathologist for signs of destruction, or change in the pattern, of the tissue—both indications of the presence of cancer.

Elizabeth had to wait a week for the results of the tests. Those seven days were difficult for the entire family. Elizabeth could not sleep, her milk began to dry up and the baby, sensing tension, became irritable and unsettled. Far from being supportive, John quietly resented the quick disintegration of his family's safe and happy routine. Now head of the pathology unit in the second largest hospital in Melbourne, he found it difficult to give up his responsibilities at work in order to fulfil his quickly burgeoning responsibilities at home. Home had always been in the capable hands of Elizabeth.

The results of the biopsy, conveyed over the phone, did little to ease the situation—indecisive. The lump did not appear to be cancer but there was no guarantee. A wider incision and surgical removal of more tissue was recommended. Elizabeth called on all her family traditions of Methodist self-reliance to cope. Her young family needed her alive and she silently promised herself that she would survive.

Elizabeth's next biopsy was known as an incisional biopsy, which

biopsy removal of a piece of tissue from the body for examination

involved the removal of a larger section, or wedge, of breast tissue. The wedge was then thinly shaved, stained with dye, set in paraffin and examined under a microscope. The medical pathologist studied the magnified sample for changes in the pattern of the tissue, or destruction of the tissue, and then made a judgment.

While this procedure is straightforward, the diagnosis can be very difficult. Sometimes an infection in the area will change the pattern of the tissue. Sometimes, if the woman is breastfeeding, or menstruating, the tissues will be affected. A benign tumour can also seem very much like a malignant tumour during initial testing. Unfortunately, Elizabeth fell into the category of 'difficult to diagnose'.

Again, the biopsy presented a dilemma: cancer could not be absolutely excluded. After several conferences between the surgeon, the radiation **oncologist** and the medical oncologist (specialising in **chemotherapy**) and numerous counselling sessions between the surgeon and Elizabeth, the recommendation was that Elizabeth have a frozen section. If the frozen section results showed that the lump was malignant (cancerous) it would be followed by a radical mastectomy. The oncologist explained that a frozen section was the examination of tissue removed from around the lump, and from the lump itself. It was frozen, sliced and examined while the patient remained under anaesthetic. If the analysis showed an increase in the amount of tissue damage, compared with the previous biopsy, it would be concluded that the lump was a malignant tumour and the surgeon would operate immediately.

Sometimes, surgeons will choose to stage the process. They will await the results of the frozen section and then perform surgery a few days later. This 'two-stage' process allows the woman time to deal with the results and prepare herself for any subsequent surgery. Elizabeth chose the 'one-stage' process. If the diagnosis was that the lump was malignant, she would undergo an immediate radical mastectomy—the removal of the whole breast, the nipple, the lymph nodes under the arm and some chest muscle.*

After the long, drawn out process of testing, waiting and retesting

---

oncologist a doctor who specialises in cancer
chemotherapy the use of chemicals and pharmaceuticals to combat cancer

Elizabeth wanted it to be over as quickly as possible, hence her 'one-stage' decision. She had learned that, if malignant, the cancer would spread rapidly and could be fatal. She had also discovered that breast cancer ran in families, and her mother's sister had died of breast cancer. Before the operation had even begun, Elizabeth had resigned herself to the probability that she would lose a breast.

Elizabeth's surgery began with the local removal of what remained of the small lump and some of the surrounding tissue. The tissues and drainage system were examined while she remained under anaesthetic. The frozen sections revealed malignant cells which had spread to her left armpit, the left axilla. Unlike the original tissue specimens, the frozen sections were clearly cancerous. Because the cancer had spread as far as the axilla the surgeons decided a radical mastectomy was necessary.

When Elizabeth woke up after the operation she felt sick, dopey and disoriented. The nausea passed after 24 hours and was replaced by a dull pain across her chest and under her left arm. To counteract the pain she was given a regular dosage of 'painkilling' tablets and injections. The next five days were devoted to improving Elizabeth's physical strength. Once she was able to feed herself, the drip supplying her with vital intravenous fluids (salt, potassium, water) was removed from her left foot. She found eating difficult so the nurses gave her easily consumable and digestible foods such as soup, pureed fruit, jelly and juice.

The surgical dressing over her wound remained in place for these five recuperation days—the time needed for primary healing to take place. On the sixth day, one of the nurses in Elizabeth's surgical ward unwrapped the bandages in order to clean the wound and check that it was healing correctly. There were some areas of infection around the lower section of the scar, indicated by redness around the stitching and the presence of weeping, or pus. The entire wound, with special attention to the infected area, was cleaned with antiseptic and then brushed down with local antibiotic powder. It was then rebandaged with a clean dressing.

The wound was dressed every two days and throughout every dressing Elizabeth turned her head away so as not to have to look at her chest. Had she looked down she would have seen a long scar starting 5 centimetres below her collarbone and running all the way down her chest to a point in line with her sternum. This was joined by another scar, starting from where her breast had been to a point just under her armpit. Because the removal of the breast meant that there was inadequate skin to cover the rib cage a skin graft had been taken (12 × 15 centimetres) from her inner leg to make up the difference. The wounds had been rejoined, and the skin graft attached with wide stitches, each tied in the middle, using nylon thread and a curved surgical needle. The large stitches and big knots, sewed unevenly down her front, made it look as if Elizabeth had been stitched up by an overgrown and rather clumsy child.

As the days passed, Elizabeth grew stronger and began to adjust to her new, postoperative body. With the firm support of the ward nurses, whose responsibility it was to teach Elizabeth how to care for herself once she returned home, Elizabeth started to observe, and then help with, their careful cleaning and rebandaging work. Once she had recovered from her initial shock, Elizabeth viewed her body with a quiet detachment; the slowly healing scars seemed to belong to someone else, someone who was very ill and fragile. Elizabeth's subconscious seemed to decide that physical recovery should come first. Once that was achieved she would begin to deal with, and hopefully accept, her loss.

Late one night an older nurse sat beside Elizabeth and held her hand. She did not speak, just offered a soft smile. Elizabeth, in a haze of sleep and discomfort, felt the warmth of the nurse's smile and imagined it was her mother sitting by her bed, as she used to when she was little, and a tiny bit frightened, during Dunolly's dark winter nights. Elizabeth felt comforted by this warm figure who cared so much about her, but it left her with a sense of overwhelming sadness that carried through into the dreams of her sleep.

After ten days the wounds had healed sufficiently to allow

Elizabeth to return home. As she was driven through the familiar streets of Hawthorn she confided to John: 'I'm not glad about what I've lost, or happy about what I've been through, but I think I probably would have done anything to get rid of that awful feeling inside. I kept imagining that a crab was eating away at the inside of my breast.'

In a way Elizabeth wasn't allowed to let that feeling go away. The treatment of breast cancer isn't limited to surgery. To destroy any remaining cancer cells, and to help prevent recurrence of the cancer, a follow-up program begins soon after surgery, once the patient has the strength to deal with the therapy. Before Elizabeth's mastectomy her medical oncologist and radiation oncologist, using information gleaned from the biopsies and the frozen section, worked together to plan a treatment for Elizabeth based on the size of her cancer and its level of **aggressiveness**.

Trial radiotherapy treatments indicated that Elizabeth's normal tissue had suffered relatively little damage in comparison with the cancerous tissue—it was the first positive news she had received. So it was decided that Elizabeth would begin a six week program involving five doses per week at the hospital's radiation oncology department. The success of such treatment would depend on the inherent difference in sensitivity to the radiation between normal tissue and cancerous tissue.

Elizabeth visited the radiation oncology department five days a week. Although she often had to wait hours for her treatment the actual therapy took only three minutes. She would lie on a bed under the machine, while the radiographer delivered a beam of radiation to her body. High-energy electromagnetic radiation, a type of focused X-ray, was used. In order to lessen normal tissue damage the beam was directed from a series of different angles.

Most people know of the awful side effects of radiation therapy. Elizabeth, who had just begun to feel that she was recovering from the trauma of surgery, once again found herself battling with her body. She had been told that most people managed to function

---

aggressiveness how quickly a cancer spreads

normally at home throughout the therapy, but after daily bouts of nausea and vomiting, coupled with extreme fatigue, she began to consider this some sort of nasty medical joke. Mrs Sutherland, who had been staying with her daughter's family for nearly two months, found herself running the household and playing mother to Elizabeth's children. John, who seemed to be finding it harder to accept the reality of the situation than anyone else in the family, finally decided to cut back on his work hours and began to accompany Elizabeth into the clinic for her almost daily therapy.

As often happens with radiation therapy patients, Elizabeth lost her appetite. As the weeks passed she began to lose weight from her already frail frame. Following the doctor's advice she tried to build up her energy by eating small snacks throughout the day, rather than the big meals she found so difficult to digest. This helped a little and Elizabeth found herself able to reinvolve herself in the day-to-day activities of the children, with special attention for Anastasia Rose, who had been so urgently weaned.

Very slowly, Elizabeth recovered her strength and after six months or so appeared to have made a full recovery. All hoped she had beaten the cancer. Because of the remaining nerves she often felt as if her breast was still there. Sometimes her left side tingled with pins and needles, an uncomfortable reminder of what she considered to be her imperfection.

Three years passed, happy years, that Elizabeth saw as an ever-growing wedge between her present self and the sickly woman of before. She devoted herself to the children and tried to strengthen her relationship with her husband. Every minute was precious: it meant a chance to listen to Anastasia chatter about preschool or watch Thomas's team win the school cricket championships. It provided an opportunity for her to impart advice to Lisa and David and gave her more time to hold her husband before they fell asleep at night.

In the early months of summer 1994, Elizabeth developed a cough, as often seems to happen when the seasons change. She couldn't shake it off and, on her third visit to the local doctor, she was referred for further tests. X-rays revealed an opaque area in the centre of the left lung. Almost certainly it was spread of the breast cancer. Further testing confirmed that the cancer had returned. Drastic measures were considered. These included the removal of Elizabeth's ovaries so as to reduce the production of oestrogen, the female hormone, which is necessary for the promotion of breast cancer. She was started on a program of tamoxifen, a new hormone medication, which counters the effects of the oestrogen and also directly suppresses the growth of breast cancer cells.

Elizabeth was also advised to undergo chemotherapy, a treatment of such high toxicity that those under treatment usually lose their hair and are sometimes left permanently infertile. Elizabeth felt she was clutching at straws. She had gone through this before—it didn't seem fair that she should have to do it all over again. But, with the passing of time once more her enemy, Elizabeth had no choice but to agree.

Chemotherapy involves the use of one drug, or a combination of drugs, given in cycles over a number of weeks or months, depending on the results. The drugs can be administered by tablets or injections although, because of their high volume and toxicity, Elizabeth was placed on an intravenous drip. She went into hospital every day, usually for five or six days running, where she would be hooked up to the drip for a few hours. After the cycle she would be given a 'rest period' of three or four days to allow her body to recover from the chemotherapy's side effects.

The drugs used in chemotherapeutic treatment kill a percentage of the quickly growing and susceptible cancer cells with each dose. Unfortunately, as with radiation therapy, a smaller number of healthy cells and tissue are also destroyed due to the toxic nature of the drugs. Elizabeth suffered from extreme nausea and bouts of vomiting during the periods of therapy. Despite eating very little, she had constant diarrhoea and felt tired and lethargic as a result.

During the third week of her treatment, her hair began to fall out. She lost huge clumps of hair, leaving large patchy sections all over her scalp. Vanity seemed out of place in such a serious situation, but

Elizabeth felt this 'last straw' was going to break her. John, sensing her fragility, tried to keep her in good spirits. After an afternoon spent shopping Elizabeth, outfitted in a new silk dress and matching scarf, which covered a newly shaved head, was escorted by John to the only French restaurant in Melbourne. For one very special evening Elizabeth felt part of the world again.

Despite minor improvements, the chemotherapy never really helped Elizabeth make much progress. Eventually, the treatment was stopped for fear it would kill her before the breast cancer did. Her weight continued to decline and it became obvious that any treament she received from then on should be purely palliative (i.e. care aimed at keeping the patient comfortable rather than seeking improvement in the underlying condition). Elizabeth did not cry when the doctors told her what she already knew—that the cancer had spread throughout her body and there was nothing more they could do. Not knowing how long she had to live, Elizabeth seemed to find freedom in the knowledge that her mortality would soon be realised. She discussed with John where she would like to be buried and they decided it should be at Hawthorn cemetery, as close as possible to the place they started their life and family together. Two plots were purchased so that one day John would be able to lie beside her.

For each of her children she made a photograph album, put together from the family collection. She covered the front of each with an enlarged photo of the family and a carefully stencilled print of their name. Beginning with their earliest baby photo she compiled their lives: through photos of their birthdays, first days at school, photos playing sport and together on family holidays, photos with aunts and uncles and cousins and photos just of them and their mum. Once finished, they were put all together on a specially labelled shelf in the living room. Elizabeth found it was the hardest thing she had ever done.

When Elizabeth died, she slipped away so quietly and peacefully it was some minutes before John realised she had gone. She had said goodbye to each of her children, in turn, taking extra time to tell

Thomas and Lisa to look after their father and help with the little ones. She was able to do little more than hold David and Anastasia as close to her as possible as they lay on either side of her.

All the children had returned to their own beds and were asleep when she passed away. Only John was with her, half asleep and holding her hand. When he woke in the early hours of the morning and realised she had gone he wasn't sure what he was supposed to do.

*Radical mastectomies have become far less common and doctors now prefer a more multimodal approach—a combination of less radical surgery, radiation therapy and chemotherapy. In the early 1980s, however, complete removal of breast and breast area was the most common form of breast cancer treatment. These days, simple lumpectomy is the preferred approach for early breast cancer, provided there is no spread to the axilla or elsewhere.[1]

what is breast cancer?

Breast cancer affects more women than any other form of cancer. The story of Elizabeth Sutherland is, sadly, far from unique. Approximately 43 000 US, 8000 UK and 2600 Australian and New Zealand women die of breast cancer each year— almost 5% of the total number of deaths among women in these countries. Nearly one in four of these deaths occurs before the age of 50 years. About 1 in 15 Western women will die as a consequence of breast cancer.

Breast cancer was a well known problem in the ancient world, probably because it afflicted women of the royal courts rather than the peasant women of the villages. This relation between status and breast cancer has continued to be recognised throughout the centuries to the current era. The first detailed descriptions of breast cancer were written on papyrus by the ancient Egyptians who were able to distinguish the features of cancer from inflammatory mastitis. Unsuccessful surgery for breast cancer was practised by both the Greeks and Romans, but in those days, without anaesthetics, the surgery must have been worse than the disease. Learned commentators such as Hippocrates advised against such radical measures. During the Renaissance period in Europe **mastectomy** again became popular, at least among surgeons; by 1650 the poor outlook for women in whom the disease had spread to the armpit was recognised. This observation remains relevant to the present day when planning treatment.

With the introduction of anaesthesia followed by blood transfusion and antibiotics over the past 100 years, surgery has become a safe procedure, including radical mastectomy where both the breast and underlying tissues are removed. But until the 1990s it is probable that such heroism by both patient and surgeon had little effect on the long-term survival of the patient. Since 1989 the outcome for women with breast cancer has improved by 1–2% each year. This appears to be due to several factors including earlier diagnosis following the introduction of **mammography** plus the use of pharmaceuticals such as tamoxifen, which suppress the cancerous process. However, as we shall repeat throughout this book, breast cancer remains a formidable problem and the development of practical strategies for its prevention is an urgent necessity.

For clues to how we might learn techniques of primary prevention in breast cancer, the medical world turns to epidemiologists. It is the work of the epidemiologist that provides one of the most important tools available in the search for the cause of breast cancer.

Epidemiology: patterns of disease

Epidemiology is a complex scientific word. It was created by modern scientists from ancient Greek, and means 'the study of the people around us'. In practice, epidemiology is the application of statistical techniques to the study of diseases in populations, as distinct from the study of individuals. Compared with open heart surgery, this is hardly the stuff of medical drama, or even a documentary, but in terms of value to the health of a community epidemiology is invaluable.

Scientists who work in this field are called epidemiologists. The work of an epidemiologist often involves years of sifting through

mammography X-ray of the breast
epidemiology the study of diseases in groups of people

mountains of data, looking for a connection or pattern. It is not surprising that many epidemiologists have 'particular' personalities. The nature of their work insists that they are earnest, obsessive and dedicated to a cause that doesn't always yield results.

Epidemiologists have been responsible for the science behind many major public health developments. Our knowledge about smoking and lung cancer, coronary heart disease, stroke, diabetes, HIV/AIDS, cholera—and even traffic accidents—is based largely on patterns discovered through epidemiological study. Dental health was revolutionised for the modern generation when water supplies were fluoridated—an action based on epidemiological studies.

However, developments based on epidemiology alone rarely provide sufficient evidence on which to base a major public health program. Additional evidence is required to confirm the clues offered by epidemiology. This may come from experiments that involve animals or humans, or from **pilot interventions**, such as giving fluoride to one community and not to another and then observing the differences. There are also the new techniques of molecular biology which involve the examination and development of genetic material. Despite this interreliance of epidemiology and other areas of research, in terms of public health it is the epidemiologists who have the greatest impact. Their work and contribution is discussed repeatedly throughout this book.

What is breast cancer?

Our bodies are made from a single cell, which is created from two cells—one from the sperm and one from the ovum. The single cell therefore contains genetic material from two people, the father and the mother. (The new developments in 'cloning', which allow for self-fertilisation and restrict genetic material to one parent only, are not relevant to the development of breast cancer.) The single fertilised cell consists of a nucleus of genetic material from both mother and father, surrounded by a sac containing nutrients. This single cell multiplies

---

pilot intervention a trial of a new treatment, to see what effects it has

many millions of times to become a **foetus** in the womb, a baby and finally an adult. Cells make up the different parts of the body—bones, muscles, brain, heart and intestines—and throughout life they replace themselves whenever necessary by continually dividing into two. This replacement occurs at different rates for different parts of the body. For example, the cells of the blood replace themselves every few weeks, whereas cells of the bones may have a life of many months. Replacement is necessary because cells become old and die, or they may be injured by trauma or toxins.

Cancerous changes in cells occur when the genetic material becomes abnormal and grows without restraint. The trigger for such cancerous changes in a particular person is generally not known. However, there are several well known and accepted initiators of such changes. Tars in tobacco smoke are classic **carcinogens**—the term for cancer initiators. Virus infections are associated with cervical cancer and some lymph cancers. Radiation, from a range of sources including the atom bomb, diagnostic X-rays and exposure to radioactive materials, can cause a variety of cancers. Excess exposure to sunlight by fair-skinned young people has resulted in a modern epidemic of **melanoma**, a cancer of the pigmented skin cells. Cells in virtually all parts of the body can become malignant or cancerous. Cancer, based on the Greek word for *crab*, is also referred to as neoplastic or 'new' growth.

The cancerous processes that lead to the creation of a thickening, or lump, in the breast are complex and their cause is largely unknown. However, such a lump has the advantage of offering an early diagnosis—in contrast to many other cancers, such as lung, prostate and colon cancer, which can remain hidden and undiagnosed for many years. An indication of a developing breast cancer is most commonly found by self-examination, or by X-ray mammography, followed by biopsy and microscopic examination of breast tissue. In

---

foetus strictly, the foetus is the product of conception to the moment of birth. At 22–24 weeks gestation, however, the foetus becomes able to live outside the womb and the term 'unborn infant' is commonly used.

carcinogen a substance that triggers cancerous changes in a cell

melanoma a cancer of the pigment-forming skin cells, caused by excessive exposure to sunlight

the scientific world such microscopic examination is called **histopathology**, another word created in modern times from ancient Greek, meaning the study of the minute structure of cells and tissues. Histopathology is the only reliable means of diagnosing breast cancer yet, as you know from the case of Elizabeth Sutherland, it is not infallible and requires the most careful judgment by an experienced and highly trained pathologist. In addition, the neoplastic tissues may not show the classic signs of malignancy and thereby inhibit the accuracy of the diagnosis.

As a further complication, there are several different types of breast cancer. Before we look at these, it is helpful to have a simple understanding of the anatomy of the breast.

Anatomy of the breast

Breasts are skin glands. During the first three months of foetal life, in both males and females, breasts begin as cells of the skin; by full term they have developed into a network of ducts without the milk-forming lobules, which do not normally appear until adolescence (although some milk-like secretions may occur from foetal breasts in response to the stimulation of maternal hormones). As the breast grows during the **peripubertal** period, fat deposits increase and ducts proliferate. Complete maturity of the breast may not occur until completion of the first full-term pregnancy. Blood vessels, nerves and lymphatic channels penetrate the breast and drain to the chest and **axilla**. These drainage systems are highly relevant to breast cancer as they provide the means for cancerous cells to spread from the breast to the immediately surrounding tissue, and eventually throughout the body. For this reason, where the cancer has spread, radical surgery is conducted. This involves the removal of skin, blood vessels, nerves and lymphatic drainage systems. The lymphatic system is the least understood of the 'support and servicing' structures of the breast. In

---

histopathology the study of the minute structure of cells and tissues; used in diagnosis
breast a modified gland of the skin
peripubertal around the time of puberty
axilla armpit

simple terms the **lymph** is the clear fluid that can be squeezed from a small wound. The main role of lymph is to work as part of the defence system of the body against infection and damage.

The breast can be readily moved over the surface of the chest but, because it is not completely separate, cancer of the breast is able to spread into the chest tissues. This lack of separation is the basis for the practice of radical mastectomy, as performed on Elizabeth Sutherland.

There are eight or more main breast ducts which spread back, into the breast, in a branching network much like a tree. The ends of these ducts become very small and frond-like and these form the basic milk secretory units and cells. About 90% of breast cancers begin in the linings of the breast ducts. Most of the remaining 10% of breast cancers appear to arise in the lining of the milk-producing units. Rare breast cancers may arise in other sections of the breast tissue, such as the connective tissue that supports the structure of the breast. The sites in the breast of the two main types of breast cancer are shown in Figure 2.1.

Figure 2.1 The sites in the breast of the two main types of breast cancer: about 90% of breast cancers arise in the linings of the milk ducts, about 10% in the linings of the milk-producing units.

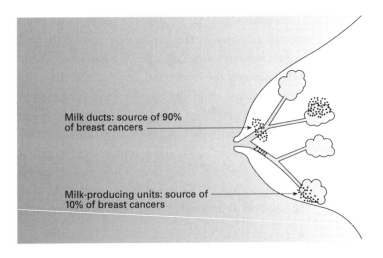

Milk ducts: source of 90% of breast cancers

Milk-producing units: source of 10% of breast cancers

---

lymph a clear fluid that circulates throughout the body and works against infection

The most important distinction is not the origin of the cancer but whether or not the cancer is **invasive** (i.e. the cancer has already spread, or is highly likely to). The histopathologist can assess this by observing the characteristics of the breast cancer cells, which can be clearly seen with a modestly powered microscope. In general, if malignant cells have the appearance of near normal cells they are less likely to spread than if they are **undifferentiated**, and do not have the appearance of normal cells. While the exact site or source of neoplastic breast cells cannot be determined, there are several accepted types of breast cancers. It is crucially important for the doctor to know what sort of breast cancer it is, as the type of cancer will determine how the cancer will develop and the most suitable plan of treatment.

The fact that breast cancer is not a single disease, and may or may not be invasive, complicates both detection and treatment. It is thought that a single breast cancer cell will double, on average, every 100–180 days. By the time a small tumour can be felt it is usually 1 centimetre in diameter and has probably been growing for 5–7 years. X-ray mammography can accelerate this detection by 1–2 years, which has been shown to be of benefit in survival terms.

Although breast cancer can spread through the blood vessels, the most dangerous spread is through the **lymphatic system**. If spread has occurred to the lymphatic system under the armpits (axillae) survival rates plummet by nearly 50%.

The technical term for the spreading of cancer is **metastasis** and, sadly, some breast cancers spread before there is even a sign of a lump in the breast. These cancers may not even be detectable by mammography. The opposite can also be the case: breast cancers can grow quite large inside the breast without ever spreading.

There are advantages to the early detection of cancer, but early detection cannot guarantee a good outlook as this also depends on a

---

invasive cancer one that invades, or spreads into, adjacent tissues
undifferentiated cancer one made up of primitive, or non-specialised, cells; such cancers are
often fast growing and potentially lethal
lymphatic system carries lymph, and forms part of the body's defence system
metastasis the spreading of a cancer

range of factors outside human influence. These factors include the nature of the cancer itself and the immune response of the body.

Breast tissue 'hormone receptors'

Over 100 years ago, in 1896, a doctor called GT Beatson noted that breast cancers in women grew at different rates in different women. While it soon became known that, in part, these differences were due to hormonal influences, not until 1961 was it shown that the breast cancer tissues themselves had differing responses to changes in hormone levels. It is now known that about half of all breast cancer tissues taken by surgical biopsy have what are termed 'oestrogen receptors'. This means there are special **proteins** (the building blocks of all tissues) in the cancer tissues which combine with or absorb circulating hormones and thereby alter the influence of these hormones. This knowledge is highly relevant for women who have been diagnosed with breast cancer as those who have such receptors are much more responsive to treatment by hormone manipulation. This knowledge also demonstrates that there are substantial differences in the types of breast cancer.

Current experimental research in animals has shown that oestrogen receptors are present very early in the foetal life of babies and that dietary fat consumed by pregnant mice and rats can influence the oestrogen receptor status in breast tissue of their female offspring.[1] This may influence subsequent breast cancer risk.

These observations also show just how complex the search for the cause of breast cancer has become!

Age distribution of patients with breast cancer

There are two peaks in the age distribution of breast cancer. About one in four breast cancer cases occurs in the first peak—the 45–49 year age group—and about three in four cases occur in the second peak—the 65–75 year age group. The remaining cases tend to fall

---

proteins the building blocks of all tissues

between these two peaks. This age distribution was recognised as early as 1930 by the German scientist Von Pirquet and confirmed by Dr F de Waard of the Netherlands in 1963.[2] De Waard remains as one of the major contributors to our understanding of breast cancer. This book includes other references to his work, in particular his hypothesis, developed in conjunction with the Greek epidemiologist Dimitrios Trichopoulos in 1988, that our diets in childhood influence the subsequent risk of breast cancer.

The observation concerning the breast cancer peaks has not led to any useful insights except to illustrate the importance of breast cancer as a cause of death in middle-aged women. With respect to Western women in the 35–54 year age group, breast cancer is the single most frequent cause of death.

The reason for the two breast cancer peaks is not known but they may be associated with the differing sex hormone patterns experienced by women during their life cycle. Prior to menopause the predominant source of oestrogens is the ovary. After menopause, the source shifts to the adrenal glands, which are situated on top of the kidneys, and to fat deposits situated throughout the body. The adrenal glands appear to secrete greater amounts of these oestrogens if there is plenty of body fat. In accord with this hypothesis, de Waard duly confirmed that there was no increase in breast cancer risk among overweight premenopausal women (who still have their oestrogen supplied by the ovaries) but there was an increased risk among those women who were overweight *after* the menopause (when the oestrogen is supplied from the adrenal glands and fat deposits). The observation that excess weight in premenopausal women is not a risk factor for breast cancer has been tested repeatedly and has been accepted as proven.[3–5]

There is an additional observation that is relevant to the search for a cause of breast cancer. This is that, although the **incidence** of breast cancer continues to rise after menopause, this rise is at a lower rate than for virtually all other forms of cancer. The implication is that breast cancer is hormone-dependent (in contrast to most other

---

incidence the extent of occurrence of a disease in a given population cancers, such as lung cancer); thus, as the level of sex hormones (such as oestrogens) falls after the menopause, the expected increase in breast cancer also falls.

Breast cancer is a complex disease and there can be no certainty about why an overweight woman should or should not develop breast cancer. All that is known is that being overweight *before* menopause is *not* a risk factor.

For older postmenopausal women who are overweight, the increase in risk is thought to be around 25%.[4] It seems possible that the rate of excess weight gain may be influential. If excess weight gain is *rapid* after the menopause, then risk of breast cancer increases. This observation is not proven but appears likely. We explore this issue more fully in Chapter 6 as weight is a risk factor for breast cancer that we can do something about.

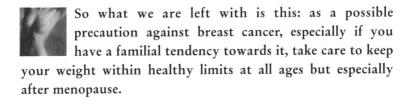 So what we are left with is this: as a possible precaution against breast cancer, especially if you have a familial tendency towards it, take care to keep your weight within healthy limits at all ages but especially after menopause.

Breast cancer and families

While **genetics** has been a strongly suspected risk factor for breast cancer, it has been difficult to differentiate between genetic and environmental factors. Family members tend to eat the same food, have similar levels of education and intelligence and similar good and bad habits, such as being 'into' sports or excessively sedentary, big drinkers or teetotallers. This makes it difficult to determine whether the prevalence of breast cancer within a family is the result of lifestyle or because of genetics. Estimates of the proportion of women with a genetic susceptibility to breast cancer have varied widely over the years from 2–20%.

genetics heredity

The latest research suggests strongly that the early work overestimated the proportion of **familial** or genetically based breast cancer.[6] In American women it seems probable that the proportion of breast cancers that are associated with a directly inherited susceptibility is about 5%. These estimates have been made from the enormous US-based research program known as *The Nurses Health Study.*[7,8]

In a brilliant piece of detective work, Jeff Hall and colleagues[6] from the School of Public Health, University of California in Berkeley, showed in 1990 that there is a breast cancer susceptibility gene located on a specific chromosome (the genetic material in every cell of the body). They further showed that this gene was confined to families who developed breast cancer before the age of 46 years. This finding has been confirmed by others and this particular breast cancer is now known as BRCA1. There have also been identified some very rare genes which carry an increased susceptibility for breast cancer. It must be noted that these breast cancer genes are carried by very few women, maybe less than 1% of all women.

These issues are well illustrated by Elizabeth Sutherland's niece, Mary. At age 31, she was concerned that she may have inherited a familial tendency towards breast cancer. The great difficulty was to separate environmental factors from possible genetic factors. The niece was well educated, well fed, took little exercise, drank alcohol moderately and had not had a baby, all of which were characteristic of her family and all of which are known risk factors for breast cancer. Genetic tests (which are expensive) were performed on Mary and were negative. Because such tests cannot exclude all genetic types of breast cancer, no guarantees could be given that she had absolutely no risk of genetic inheritance of breast cancer. The final result for the niece was that no definite answers could be given and that the most appropriate action would be to have regular mammograms.

---

familial affecting several members of the same family (but not necessarily genetic)

The Nurses Health Study

The Nurses Health Study was developed during the early 1970s by the Harvard School of Public Health in Boston, Massachusetts, and is led by the 'Who's Who' of US breast cancer epidemiologists, Frank Speizer. Speizer is the physician who, with his colleagues, originally conceived of the study and set up a small pilot program to demonstrate its potential value to funding authorities. Over the years, as the project has produced ever more sophisticated results, Speizer has kept a modest profile, content to have his name at the end or in the middle of the list of authors and rarely in the prized leading position. In the scientific world, authorship means finance, fame and international speaking tours, none of which has proved attractive to Frank. He has been perfectly happy supporting the project and encouraging others. The leadership role has been largely taken over by an engaging, somewhat controversial workaholic physician/epidemiologist, Walter Willett.

The study, which costs about $1 000 000 each year, has been worth every cent. Originally funded to determine whether there were any links between oral contraceptives and cancer, the study has expanded to include a broad range of women's health problems. In any such study the big problem is to identify participants who will stay with the program for 20 or more years and who will conscientiously answer the questions truthfully and accurately. Initially, the female spouses of US physicians were approached because Speizer and colleagues believed they would understand the objectives of the study and fulfil the long-term requirements. This did not happen as expected and there were many early withdrawals from the study. Nurses were then chosen as the subjects for study because they were considered most likely to give a high response rate. (Unless most participants respond, such studies rapidly lose their reliability.) Thanks to these US nurses and the diligence of the research team, the response rate has been over 90% for more than 20 years— quite remarkable.

The Nurses Health Study has provided reliable information with respect to US and similar Western women about diet, breastfeeding, height, weight, oral contraception, hormone replacement therapy, diabetes, and a range of cancers. Indeed, this book would not have been possible without the information created by this amazing study.

The Nurses Health Study has shown that the risk of breast cancer is approximately doubled among women whose mothers had breast cancer diagnosed before the age of 40 years, or who have a sister with breast cancer. The risk is elevated even for those whose mothers were diagnosed with breast cancer at the age of 70 years or older. These risks do not change for US women with obesity or other risk factors.

More recent findings from *The Nurses Health Study* have shown that, for women with a mother/sister history of the disease, the accepted reproductive risk factors for breast cancer are different from women without a family history.[8] In particular, for women with a strong family history of breast cancer there is little protection from the known reducers of risk, such as late age at **menarche** (onset of puberty) and early age at first birth. Thus a woman whose periods begin late and who has her first baby at, say, age 22 years, but who has a strong family history of breast cancer, does not enjoy the protection from breast cancer that these two factors usually offer. There are no known reasons for these observations. Unfortunately, they apply to Elizabeth Sutherland, whose mother's sister died of breast cancer.

In the absence of similar studies in countries such as Japan and China, it is difficult to be sure of the degree of influence that genetics has in Asian and other populations. Limited studies suggest that the proportions of familial breast cancer are likely to be of the same order as among the US population.[9,10]

Environmental factors

The rates of breast cancer vary greatly in different populations.[11]

The rates in the United States, Europe and Australia are up to ten times greater than in parts of rural Japan and China. Studies of migrants from these countries have shown that these differences are not due to genetics or different reproductive practices. Women who migrate from developing to developed countries experience an

---

menarche onset of menstruation

increase in breast cancer and, over several generations, their risk of breast cancer nearly matches that of the host country. These observations have led to a massive international research interest, but with little result. However, there are some clues.

Over 25 years ago, a tireless research worker in this field, Brian MacMahon of Harvard, showed that not only were there differences in breast cancer risks between populations, there were striking differences in the age profiles.[12] Where breast cancer rates are high, risk continues throughout life; where the risk is low—as in Japan—the risk increases until middle life, then plateaus, and after age 50 it begins to decline. So an American woman is at increasing risk of breast cancer throughout life, whereas a Japanese woman is at low and reducing risk as she becomes older. The explanation for the difference is not known but may be related to the excess weight of many postmenopausal Western women.

Diet

Dietary variations between Asian, Mediterranean and Western populations are strongly suspected to be the cause of the differing breast cancer rates. The real mystery has been *how* diet influences the risk of breast cancer. There have been a great many studies aimed at finding a dietary link. During the 1980s a majority of studies suggested that fat was the culprit,[13,14] but later studies have not confirmed these findings.[15] However, studies of women from southern Mediterranean countries have demonstrated the possibility that consumption of olive oil may reduce the risk of breast cancer.[16,17]

Olive oil is composed mainly of unsaturated fats, unlike animal fats which are saturated. The concept of saturated and unsaturated chemicals (in this case, fats) is not easy to understand. In simple terms, *unsaturated* means that the combinations of chemicals—in the case of fats these are carbons—can accept additional chemical molecules until the whole becomes 'saturated'. Whether the substance, such as fat, is fully saturated or unsaturated affects the behaviour and characteristics of the fat. The best known and most important example is the blocking effect that saturated fats have on the coronary arteries of the heart. Unsaturated fats do not have such an effect. With breast cancer, however, the research is too limited to know for sure whether olive oil provides protection. Findings from 1998 Swedish research suggest it is monounsaturated fat that may reduce risk of breast cancer, and not the olive oil as such. Olive oil is very high in monounsaturated fats.[18]

There have been suggestions that vitamins offer protection against breast cancer. Again, there have been no consistent answers[19-22] although it seems possible that vitamin A may offer some limited protection. Fish, meat and coloured vegetables such as peas, beans, carrots and marrow contain high levels of vitamin A.

Some more clearly definable connections between diet and breast cancer have begun to emerge. The most revealing has been the realisation that almost all studies observe patterns of food consumption in adults, *not in young people*. This clue came from the observation that migrants who came to a high-risk country when they were children were at greater risk of breast cancer than their migrating parents. This observation is discussed more fully later in the book (see 'Insights from migrants', p. 49).

Reproduction

One of the earliest known features of breast cancer was that it is more common in nuns than other women.[23] The most obvious difference between these two groups is that nuns do not have children and do not breastfeed, whereas most other women do. Using this information as a starting block, Brian MacMahon furthered our understanding of the connection between reproduction and breast cancer.[24]

It is now known that breast cancer risk increases as the age at which a woman bears her first full-term child increases.[25,26] **In other words, full-term pregnancy at a young age offers substantial protection against breast cancer.**

The following information is not straightforward. Please bear with us!

Full-term pregnancy has a dual effect on risk of breast cancer: it transiently (for about three years) increases the risk after childbirth but reduces the risk in later years. Multiple **parity** reduces the risk of breast cancer by about 10% for each additional pregnancy.

If a woman has a baby before the age of 20 years she will receive the greatest amount of protection against breast cancer. A woman having a baby before the age of 30 will receive partial protection. The risk is approximately halved for pregnancy before 20, as compared with 30 years. The major protective effect appears to be limited to the first birth, but additional births add a little to the level of protection. This protection is exerted only by a full-term pregnancy and lasts throughout the woman's life span.

 The belief that breastfeeding lowers the risk of breast cancer has existed for over 50 years. This has not been confirmed by recent studies on American women[27,28] **who breastfeed for comparatively short periods, but it appears likely that prolonged breastfeeding, for 2 years or more, does convey some protection.**[9,10,29]

Age at menarche

Menarche is the formal name for the onset of menstruation. The observation that age at menarche is associated with risk of breast cancer has been consistent over many years, and among both

---

parity number of pregnancies
menarche onset of menstruation

low-risk[9,10] and high-risk breast cancer populations.[25,26,30,32] The earlier the age a female begins to menstruate, the higher the risk of breast cancer. The risk changes by approximately 5–10% for every year. The age at menarche depends largely on a girl's weight, which in turn is very dependent on diet and exercise.[33]

Age at menopause

The weight of evidence suggests that women with late natural menopause have increased risk of breast cancer.[25,26,32] Women with natural menopause at age 55 years or older have approximately twice the risk of those whose menopause occurs naturally before age 45 years.

As with menarche, the determinants of the age at menopause are not clear but international variations are compatible with diet again being a major influence. Well fed Western women have a later menopause than less well fed Asian women.[9,10]

The ovaries and breast cancer

Not only do the ovaries produce life, in the form of eggs, or ova, they also produce female sex hormones, mainly oestrogens. Oestrogens are a necessary ingredient for the development of breast cancer. Evidence of this has been given repeatedly—when the ovaries are surgically removed the risk of breast cancer falls.[34,35] Among women who have undergone surgical removal of the ovaries, it has been found that younger women gain the greatest benefit in terms of lower risk of breast cancer. If a woman has the surgery before the age of 35 the reduction in risk is 70%. Even 40 years later, among women beyond the age of 75 years, the risk of breast cancer is halved for those women who had the ovaries removed before they were 45 years old.

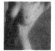 **The strongest evidence supporting the major role sex hormones play in breast cancer is the fact that the risk of breast cancer is over 100 times greater in women than in men.**

There is additional evidence to implicate the role of sex hormones in breast cancer. There is considerable, but to some extent conflicting, evidence to support the notion that women who have higher than normal sex hormone blood levels are at increased risk of breast cancer. This circumstantial evidence (evidence which implies an association but may not be the actual cause) includes the observation that Chinese adult women have less than half the blood levels of sex hormones than British or US women.[36,37] The reason why women have different levels of sex hormones in their bodies is complex but diet appears to be the most influential factor.[38]

The complexity of the issue is shown by the observation that women who consume diets that are high in energy and fats also have high sex hormone levels, and such women are at higher risk of breast cancer. However, careful studies have failed to show any direct link between consumption of fat by adult women and breast cancer! We can only speculate about the reasons for these conflicting observations. It could be that different types of fat—say, animal fats as compared with vegetable-sourced fats—act in different ways. There is some evidence to suggest this could well be true.

Socioeconomic status and health

For many years it has been recognised that women of higher socioeconomic status (social class) are at greater risk of breast cancer than women from the same population who are of low socioeconomic status.[39-41] It has been suggested that these differences reflect different reproductive patterns, such as age at first birth, age at menarche and number of children. However, as will be shown, there are other more

circumstantial evidence implies an association, but may not be the *cause*

probable reasons—such as different dietary patterns among different social classes, whereby socioeconomic status is an indication of the standard of nutrition during pregnancy and childhood.

In summary, the generally accepted risk factors for breast cancer are:

1 Being female—breast cancer is more than 100 times more common in women than in men.
2 Being born in a Western country—breast cancer is up to ten times more common in the United States than in parts of rural China.
3 Being older—breast cancer does occur among young women, but is three times more common in women over the age of 50 years.
4 The age at menarche and menopause influences the risk of breast cancer. The younger the age at menarche the greater the risk; the older the age at menopause the greater the risk.
5 The age at first full-term pregnancy influences the risk, which is nearly double for women aged 30 years or over as compared with women aged 20 years or less.
6 There is a small (about 5%) but confirmed genetic factor for susceptibility to risk of breast cancer. Some argue that there is a familial trend for up to 15% of all women who have breast cancer.

Nothing can be done about being female and old, it is difficult to avoid a familial trend, and few Western and modern Asian women are going to get pregnant at 19 years of age as a measure against breast cancer. Is the prevention of breast cancer thus an impossible task?

Diagnosis and survival

The diagnosis of breast cancer is made initially by one of three methods:
1 by self-examination of the breast
2 by clinical examination—that is, by a doctor or other health

professional who may examine the breast during a special 'check-up' or during attendance at a clinic for an unrelated purpose such as influenza

3 by mammography, a special X-ray examination whose purpose is to detect breast cancer.

This initial diagnosis has to be confirmed by a microscopic examination of the surgically removed lump or tissue.

It has been shown that patients whose breast cancer is detected by mammography have an approximately 10% better chance of survival after 5 years and a 20% better chance of survival after 10 years than patients detected by the other methods.[42] The reason for this is that women with invasive breast cancer detected by mammography have smaller tumours and the tumour is less likely to have spread. Detailed consideration is given to the method of breast self-examination in Chapter 13.

The influence of mammography on the early diagnosis of breast cancer has been greater than breast self-examination, mainly because breast cancer can be detected at an earlier stage by mammography than by breast self-examination. However, mammography is not perfect although it can pick up about 90% of all early breast cancers. Hormone replacement therapy can increase the density of breast tissue and thereby obscure the clarity of the image needed to diagnose breast cancer by mammography. In addition, some breast cancers can develop rapidly between mammography examinations, and breast self-examination may detect such cancers before a yearly or two-yearly mammography.

Despite the higher rate of survival, however, breast cancer remains a lethal disease.[43] About 15% of those women who contract breast cancer will die within two years of the diagnosis. Ten years after diagnosis approximately half will have died, and 55–60% die after 15 years. The longer they live, the better their chance of survival. Contrary to expectations based on observations of other cancers, those women diagnosed at younger ages have a better outlook than others. Death rates due to breast cancer in women in premenopausal age groups are 1–2% per year, but rise to over 5% per year for women diagnosed over 75 years of age.

This is all extremely gloomy, but there is some good news, too. Recent experiences have shown that mammography for women of all ages reduces deaths due to breast cancer by some 30% over a ten year period.[44] There is a lesser (13%) reduction in women aged 40–50 years who, despite the comments above, may experience a higher proportion of breast cancers that progress rapidly.

United States death rates for white women increased slightly during the 1980s but have fallen by approximately 2% each year among all age groups since 1989.[45] These falls have been matched by similar falls in the UK, Australia and Canada.[46,47] This exciting news is probably due to a combination of early detection by mammography plus radiotherapy and chemotherapy. The pharmaceutical, tamoxifen, is credited with the recent improvement in **outcome** for breast cancer in the UK and may have had an influence in the US.[46] Some commentators have suggested using tamoxifen as a primary prevention measure in high-risk females. This is entirely reasonable for women who, for example, have breast cancer in one breast and are therefore at increased risk of developing breast cancer in the other breast. Clearly, the gains may outweigh the risks. But the use of tamoxifen and similar chemicals to prevent breast cancer is an inappropriate approach when applied to whole communities of normal women, because of an increased risk of **endometrial** (lining of the womb) **cancer** and possible adverse effects on the liver.

There has also been a substantial decline in the numbers of women who have spread of the cancer to the **axilla** at the time of diagnosis, and this is almost certainly due to mammography. Diagnosis before such spread is crucial as the average period of survival after diagnosis of metastatic disease (spread) is only 18–24 months, although this varies widely between patients.[45]

---

outcome results of treatment
endometrial cancer cancer of the lining of the womb
axilla armpit

During the past decade there has been substantial progress in the search for a 'cure' for breast and other cancers. However, it must be emphasised that almost all the work has been on experimental animals and it will take many years for the necessary studies to be carried out on humans. In addition, what works in animals often does not work in humans.

Among this new work is that of Judah Folkman from the Children's Hospital in Boston.[48] Folkman is credited with pursuing the concept of stopping the growth of blood vessels which supply nutrients to cancerous growths. He based this concept on the common observation that, when a large tumour is surgically removed from a patient, the removal seems to set off the growth of many smaller tumours. Therefore, he hypothesised that the original tumour may produce a substance that inhibits the growth of other tumours that would have competed for survival with the original tumour. After 15 years work with colleague Michael O'Reilly, Folkman was able to identify a naturally occurring protein which had the ability to stop a tumour from growing. They then found another natural protein which, when used in combination with the first protein, actually caused the tumour to disappear. These proteins worked as hypothesised by preventing or destroying the blood vessels supplying the tumours.

However, these studies have all been conducted in mice and, as Folkman has said, 'If you have cancer and you're a mouse, we can take good care of you.'[49] His implication is that these results may or may not apply in humans. It will take many years to find out.

While Folkman's **anti-angiogenesis** (a process that blocks the formation of new blood supplies to cancer tumours) approach is the most dramatic, there are several promising alternatives:

■ the use of chemicals to confine the growth of cancers to one place and prevent their spread

■ the development of anti-cancer vaccines from the cancer tumours themselves

■ the development of substances that counter the effect of sex

---

anti-angiogenesis a process blocking new blood supplies to cancer tumours

hormones on cancers—tamoxifen and raloxifene are examples in the case of breast cancer

■ the development of viruses that can carry tumour-suppressing genes

■ the manufacture of antibodies that stop tumours from growing.

Despite this substantial progress, breast cancer remains a major problem and a potentially fatal disease. It would obviously be much better if a cause for breast cancer were found and prevention strategies were developed.

3

breasts and their meaning

Breast cancer is of great concern to many women. Breast cancer is of more concern than coronary heart disease, stroke and diabetes, all of which are more likely to cause death and disability. Why is it so?

This is a very practical question because there is hard evidence to show that, if women are offered specific ways of reducing breast cancer, they are far more likely to act than if they are confronting circulatory disorders.[1,2]

The powerful description below, by author Helen Garner, is of a photograph of a rebellious young student at the University of Melbourne. It is obvious to all that her bosom is of vastly greater significance to her than her circulatory system.

'The first impression it creates is one of shining. Then one notices the amount of flesh that is permitted to shine. The gaze, whether one is male or female, drops like a stone from top to bottom of this photo, then travels slowly up. She is wearing a dark, strapless evening dress, out of which the double mass of her splendid bosom—the only possible word for it—is bursting. Her face and shoulders are tanned, her eyes are glowing, her dark-lipped, enormous mouth is split wide in a frank grin, showing perfect teeth. Her face is so dazzling that her hair, worn up and back except for one free curl over her right eye, is only a shadow. It is impossible not to be moved by her daring beauty. She is a woman in the full glory of her youth, as joyful as a goddess, elated by her own careless authority and power.'[3]

The bosom is the most common feature of mass marketing. Breasts have become a selling point, the symbol for everything desirable—beauty, youth, family, opulence. In Western societies and to a lesser, but more subtle, extent in the East, there is a constant bombardment with the image of breasts. Open up a weekend magazine and there they are, firm but sleek, ensconced in a designer dress; watch television and there they are again, peeping up over the dashboard of the latest Japanese car. They are on the back of buses, bouncing about in holiday brochures, they dominate the movies—eat an icecream and you can be sure the brand you chose once nestled lovingly in some bountiful cleavage.

You can't get much more 'in your face' than the ten tonne billboard breasts, the advertising executive's thankful offering to the gods. Is it any wonder that their monstrous scale and generous exposure is the cause of so much motorist havoc? Can you blame the awe-struck bloke in the truck behind you for plowing straight into the back of your zippy small car—the one you bought so you could have breasts like hers? There seems to be no level of breast exposure that is deemed as overkill. Like teenagers who believe they invented sex, advertisers seem to think that they created breasts.

Fortunately for women—or perhaps unfortunately—the advertising agencies didn't create them, and the world isn't full of uniformly firm, pert D-cup breasts. The reality, that breasts come in numerous shapes, sizes and colours, is probably a hard fact for a child of the television generation to come to terms with. I know that when I was pre-puberty I fully expected to be endowed one day with a pair that would make me as perfect as Cindy Crawford. I never thought it strange that two swellings, consisting largely of fat cells and tissue, whose primary function is to feed and nurture should play such an important role in the way I felt about myself.

In our society a girl's first period is treated privately; it is a quiet crossing-over into womanhood. The development of breasts, on the other hand, is a highly visible, and therefore public, signal that the half-proud, half-embarrassed owner is no longer a girl. I vividly remember my primary school years when, through observation and gossip, everyone knew which girls wore bras and what size they were. I doubt that these girls were any more mature than us but we looked up to them, as admiring as any boy. As far as we flat-chested ones were concerned, they were women. Boys treated them differently, teachers treated them more respectfully, we admired them, simply because they had breasts.

Two years later I went to the local shopping centre with a couple of girlfriends. Although still relatively unendowed we were all determined to join the ranks of 'women', so we ventured into the lingerie section of Grace Bros. I bravely asked the lady assistant where bras, 'a bit smaller than these' were, and a tangled and embarrassed hour later we were all proud owners of a bra. As far as we were concerned, we were now women—and we had the cotton-wool enhanced breasts and training bra to prove it.

Although my breasts got bigger they were never the fulsome beauties I was hoping for. You didn't need to be a genius, or even sexually experienced, to know that big breasts were good and small breasts were, well, not good enough. As a girl of thirteen you understood that if you were 'well endowed' you were more attractive to the opposite sex. You also knew that, regardless of size, you had to be mindful of how you displayed them; if you showed too much, people might think you were slutty, so you had to be pretty careful. If you were small or flat-chested you were probably a lot smarter, and probably a bit more manly as well, two things that weren't going to score you any points.

It is not only in our generation that breasts have been attributed with so much importance. I recently borrowed a book from our local library called *The Human Figure*. A more appropriate title would have been *Breasts through History*—it was the sort of book that school librarians are forever trying to hide from their sharp-eyed, anatomically-obsessed fifth graders. Although the artists of the last couple of millennia did not plunder the image of the breast for sinfully economic reasons, breasts are as regularly featured and devotedly focused upon as the most powerful of idols.

Almost every artist depicting the human form, from Palaeolithic sculptures through to modern and contemporary art, uses the breast to denote the form as female. This observation probably comes as no great surprise to anyone—females have breasts, it's only natural that the female form is represented with them. But females also have bigger hips, fuller lips and a larger, fuller bottom than a male and, most pertinent of all, a vagina rather than a penis. In art forms, where the human body is reduced to its most essential visual components—such as in very primitive art or the pre-abstract work of artists like Picasso—the breast, whether represented by a lump or merely a line, is considered to be the clearest visual indication that the figure is a woman. One of the major differences in the physical form of male and female, the breast represents more than an anatomical feature—it is transformed into the symbol of female.

This symbol was moulded according to the aspect of female the artist wanted to emphasise. In primitive art, the female was seen primarily as the child-bearer, so their 'impression' of the female form was a figure with hugely exaggerated breasts—such as the small stone Venus of Willendorf, a squat little figure with breasts like mountain outcrops. The notion of a fertility goddess as a figure with large protruding breasts was repeated throughout history, and from continent to continent. Be it a stone carving from Ancient Greece, a terracotta figure from Mesopotamia or a wooden woman from the Ivory Coast, the concept of 'female' was synonymous with the concept of fertility, and the symbol for both of these was hugely swollen breasts.

In modern times it became clear that the female was no longer considered primarily as a reproducer or child-bearer. How was this apparent? Gone were the enormous bosoms of the primitive age, and in their place was the breast we are more accustomed to seeing in today's art—the sexy breast. No less eye-catching, the breast has been moulded into a shape that is less formidable and more erotic than that depicted in the past. Intentionally unrealistic, the modern idealised breast has evolved as the ultimate symbol of female beauty and sexuality.

As final proof of the crucial role that breasts play in the lives of modern women is the highly fashionable practice of breast augmentation. Breast augmentation involves the insertion of a silicone-based shell beneath the skin and muscles of the chest. This shell is then inflated with saline. The results vary from subtle enlargement to the grossly unreal 'superbreasts' that have become so popular among film and other stars. It is believed that more than two million American women have had their breasts augmented during the past decade.[4]

The female form, with breasts exaggerated and idealised, has become a symbol, a sign—'I am female, I am fertile, I am sexual'. Yet what happens when the symbol becomes more potent an image than the thing it is intended to symbolise? When the breast has more meaning than the woman? Perhaps this is why the issue of breast cancer attracts so much public attention, research interest and financial support. As breasts are *the* symbol of womanhood, cancer of the breast does not simply invade fat, muscle and blood vessels; such a malignancy threatens to remove our identity—as sexual, nurturing, female creatures.

Although Elizabeth Sutherland hardly fits into the busty, erotic picture that has been painted above, even the most demure and genteel of women are influenced by the constant promotion of the bosom. We can only speculate about Elizabeth's feelings at the loss of the breast that had fed and nurtured her children, consoled and aroused her husband, given her status as a woman, and finally killed her.

4

diet

International evidence on diet

Food consumption is likely to be associated in some way with risk of breast cancer. Latest indications are that food consumption patterns during pregnancy, childhood and teenage may be of special significance.

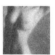 **Breast cancer is up to 6–10 times more common in Western countries than in Asian countries.**

This observation and the possible link between diet and breast cancer appears to have been first made in 1966 by AJ Lea and other workers.[1] However, it was Bruce Armstrong and Richard Doll who, in 1975, offered the first formal study that linked national diets with such patterns of breast cancer.[2]

Armstrong and Doll are epidemiologists who at the time of these studies were working from the Radcliffe Infirmary, a famous and ancient hospital in Oxford. Both fit, almost perfectly, the personality profile for that professional group. Bruce, an Australian, is quiet and serious by nature. He has the delicate appearance of a scholar, a man who spends most of his time at work in his study. Richard, now Sir

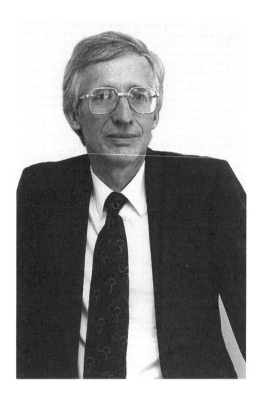

Bruce Armstrong, one of Australia's leading scientists. Together with Sir Richard Doll, of Oxford, he showed that national diets that were high in fats and energy were associated with increased rates of breast and other cancers. His work stimulated a 20 year international search for possible links between fat consumption and breast cancer.

Richard, is tall, with a backbone that lends dignity rather than stiffness, and a reserved manner that suggests a touch of intolerance. He carries his title with a confidence that suggests he was always called Sir Richard. He is recognised as the scientist who proved the link between lung cancer and tobacco. He did this by observing, for a period that was to extend for over 40 years, the difference in lung cancer rates among British doctors who gave up smoking and those who continued to smoke. He was able to show that smoking doubled the lung cancer risk.

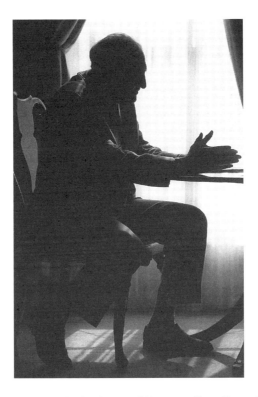

Sir Richard Doll, photographed at the age of 85 years, still working and travelling full time. Perhaps the most famous of all epidemiologists, Sir Richard was the scientist mainly responsible for proving the link between tobacco smoking and lung cancer. With Bruce Armstrong he also showed the link between national consumption of fats and energy and breast cancer.

Fats in the diet

Armstrong and Doll showed that consumption of diets high in fats and possibly animal proteins may be associated with increased risk of breast cancer. Their views were compatible with the few studies available then that showed a link between obesity and breast cancer.[3]

This information is shown in Figure 4.1. It is not easy to comprehend this mass of data but, because it is important in the search for the cause of breast cancer, it is a task worth pursuing.

Figure 4.1 shows that deaths from breast cancer, recorded as rates for every 100 000 women, vary enormously between countries. Death rates due to breast cancer are up to six times higher in the United States, the United Kingdom and other economically developed countries of Europe and Australasia compared with Japan, Korea, Hong Kong and China. These differences may be as much as tenfold when Western women are compared with women from rural areas in Asia.

Figure 4.1 Breast cancer deaths, selected countries, 1994 (age-adjusted rates per 100 000). These data show dramatically that the death rates for breast cancer vary between countries by a factor of 6 to 10. These great differences are not due to genetic inherited factors—when women migrate from countries with a low risk of breast cancer to high-risk countries, within two generations the death rate among their offspring rises to near that of the host population.

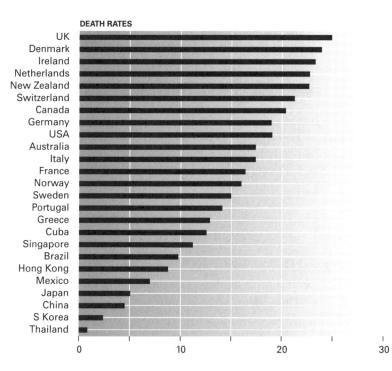

Source: World Health Organisation, World Health Statistics Annual 1995, Geneva 1996.

In most of the countries listed in Figure 4.1, the diagnosis of breast cancer is confirmed by microscopic examination of the tissues by medical pathologists. The cause-of-death certificate is collected by a central office of statistics and is considered to be reasonably accurate. To allow comparisons to be made between countries, adjustments have been made for the different ages of women living in each country (the data is said to be 'age-adjusted').

In Figure 4.2, the daily energy consumption per head of population, expressed as calories, for each country is shown for 1961/65 and compared with the death rates for 1994. In general, the higher the consumption of calories, the higher the consumption of fats and proteins. This information comes from estimates made by the United Nations Food and Agriculture Organisation based in Rome.

Figure 4.2 Breast cancer deaths and consumption of calories, selected countries, 1994 (age-adjusted death rates per 100 000; national per capita daily average consumption of calories). These data show the strong correlation between deaths due to breast cancer and consumption of energy (calories). Research shows this is not due to consumption of fats by adults. There has to be another explanation, but what is it? This unanswered question has challenged international scientists for more than two decades.

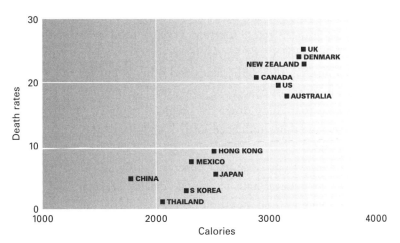

Sources: 1. World Health Organisation, World Health Statistics Annual 1995, Geneva 1996; 2. Food and Agriculture Organisation of the United Nations, Food balance tables 1994, Rome 1996.

Use of this information for epidemiological purposes has been criticised because it overestimates the amount of food consumed and also because it includes infants, women and children, who obviously eat different amounts of food from male labourers.[4] This criticism is reasonable if the purpose is to measure the consumption of food by individuals, but the use of such information for the observation of trends and for comparisons between populations has been shown to be valid.[6]

There is a serious bias in the information in Figures 4.1 and 4.2 as only those countries for which data is available are listed. Such countries are economically better developed and generally have better food supplies than the many countries that are not listed. For example, the experience of India, Pakistan and Bangladesh is not shown because the data is not available.

The data clearly demonstrates that countries (populations) with high levels of food consumption have high levels of breast cancer. However, there is another key observation to be made. It has been noticed that correlations are much greater between food consumption levels in the 1960s and breast cancer death rates in the 1990s, than between current (i.e. 1990s) food consumption levels and breast cancer rates. Current (1990s) food consumption in Hong Kong and South Korea is at similar levels to Australia, Canada, Sweden, the Netherlands and other countries and yet the deaths due to breast cancer are very low. The implication is that it is probable that diets eaten by pregnant women, children and teenagers have more influence on risk of breast cancer than diets eaten as adults.

But we need to make another observation. Breast cancer rates are increasing at a faster rate in young females in Japan and other countries where food consumption by children and teenagers increased rapidly about 30 years ago.

These observations, made in relation to Japan, apply similarly to other countries that had low food consumption patterns and low breast cancer rates in the 1960s, and where both food consumption and breast cancer rates have substantially increased. These countries include Greece, Portugal, Italy and Singapore.

These observations offer support for the view expressed above, that diets consumed in childhood, or even during pregnancy, may be influential on subsequent susceptibility to breast cancer.

It is also clear that as national diets 'improve', or increase, over the years, there is a parallel increase in breast cancer mortality rates. The word 'improve' is placed in quotation marks because diets can increase but not improve in a health sense; for example, many Western populations, who were already well fed 50 years ago, have increased their food consumption levels and, as a result, have worsened their diets by an excess consumption of fats and other foods.

Elizabeth Sutherland is only one of the millions of modern Western women who are at 6–10 times the risk of breast cancer, compared with their Asian counterparts. Her diet, high in milk, meat and cream, was very typical of economically affluent Western families of the period. Although, as observed above, fat consumed during adult life by Elizabeth was probably not associated with her breast cancer, there remains a suspicion that her diet adversely influenced events.

Insights from migrants

Some of the most revealing insights into breast cancer have come from observations of migrants. The main destinations of the great twentieth century migration movements have been countries at high risk of breast cancer—the United States, Canada, New Zealand and Australia. However, migrants as a source of information about cancer were not explored in detail until the 1960s, despite the existence of the data in the ageing files of the US Bureau of Census since 1900. As long ago as 1913, WH Davis noted and published the substantial differences in the mortality rates from cancer and other causes among foreign-born groups in Boston, but this early work attracted little attention.[6] The practice of scientists 'marketing' their work did not begin until more than half a century later.

HL Lombard and CR Doering, who worked in the US during the 1920s, were the first to provide a systematic review of cancer mortality by site (stomach, lung, prostate, breast) among migrants. They suggested that the differences in cancer patterns they observed between migrant and local citizens were due to economic and social conditions.[7]

Again the issue was neglected until DF Eastcott noted the differences in cancer mortality between migrants and native-born residents in another country of immigrants, New Zealand. The issue attracted increasing interest after the war years, culminating in the studies by William Haenszel from the US National Cancer Institute in Bethesda, Maryland.[8,9] He was the first to show that breast cancer mortality among migrants from the UK and Western European countries was similar to native-born US Caucasians, but that the rates were much lower among migrants from Italy and Poland.

Nearly 10 years later he was able to show that breast cancer in Japanese migrants to the US remained low for two generations.[9] This was in contrast to cancer of the colon in Japanese migrants which, within one generation, rose to almost equal the higher risk for US whites. These observations were to become specially significant more than 20 years later when Dimitrios Trichopoulos, an Athenian epidemiologist, developed his theories for the causation of breast cancer.

The mortality rates for most cancers among migrants gradually move away from the level found in their country of birth towards the mortality rate of the host country.[6] The increased risk of breast cancer among migrants can be dramatic, as shown by the sixfold gradient in risk of breast cancer among female migrants from rural Asia to the US, when compared with US-born Asians of two generations.[10] With respect to breast cancer among migrants from countries at low risk of breast cancer to high-risk countries (which correlate with low to high 'rich'-food-consuming countries), the rates alter according to the overall differences in the incidence of breast cancer between the originating and the host countries, the period of residence in the host country, and whether the women were born in the host country. In addition, with respect to migrants who have lived for an approximately equal period in a host country, the earlier the age of migration the higher the increase in breast cancer rates.[11]

The experience of migration from historically low-risk-of-breast-cancer countries, such as Italy and Greece, to a high-risk country like Australia provides an opportunity to examine breast cancer rates among those who migrated at an early age and those who migrated at a late age. As shown in Table 4.1, those who migrated before the age of 20 years had much higher mortality rates from premenopausal breast cancer compared with those who migrated after the age of 20 years. Although these observations need to be treated with caution because of the methods used (comparison of groups of people as compared with observing individuals over many years) to compile the information, the pattern is similar to that among young people migrating from the south to the north of Italy.[12,13]

It has also been observed that Japanese women who migrate to the United States at an early age develop higher rates of breast cancer than those who migrate at a late age but, once again, breast cancer rates for both these migrant groups is lower than for US-born Japanese.[14]

These observations are all indirect, which means that it is not the same person who is being followed from time of migration to the time of contracting breast cancer. To some extent this is a possible source of inaccuracy.

In the first study to evaluate directly the hypothesis that an early age at migration to the US exposes Asian women to Western lifestyles at a crucial age, Ziegler and his research group found the risk of breast cancer declined steadily among Asian women migrating at later ages.[10] As referred to above, these findings have since been confirmed by studies of internal Italian migrants of various ages.[12,13] Those who migrate from low- to high-income areas, and who consume richer diets as a consequence, experience greater breast cancer risk the younger the age of migration. For women who migrated after the age of 24 years, their risk of breast cancer remained at least one-third lower than those who migrated before the age of 24 years.[13]

The risk of breast cancer among Italian migrants to Australia increases according to their length of residence in Australia.[15] For Italian migrants whose duration of residence in Australia exceeds 17 years the risk of breast cancer doubles, compared with their homeland, and equals that of Australian-born Italians. As shown in Table 4.1, it is likely that most of this increase in risk occurs if migration takes place before the age of 20 years. By way of contrast, migrants to Australia from high-risk-of-breast-cancer countries, such as the United Kingdom, have high but similar risks of developing breast cancer as their compatriots remaining in the UK.

These changes in breast cancer rates among migrants from low- to high-risk countries have been associated with changes in their diets after migrating. Italians eat more bread and pasta, salami, vegetables, fish and red wine than traditional Australians. Once they migrate to Australia, they tend gradually to add more meat and fat to their traditional diets.[16] Greek immigrants, despite a strong desire to maintain their culture, also eat more meat and fat after coming to Australia.[17] It is a common pattern that migrants maintain the original cuisine of their country but enrich the diet by adding more meat and fatty foods.[18,19]

The hypothesis that nutritional experiences before the age of 20 years are relevant to subsequent risk of breast cancer is strengthened by recent large prospective studies. These studies demonstrate that fat consumption during adult life is not a risk factor for breast cancer.[20] In addition, as we have previously explored, there is compelling evidence that an early menarche increases risk by approximately 5% for each year below the age of 17 or 18 years, and that age at menarche is dependent on weight, which in turn depends mainly on nutritional experiences during childhood.[21-2]

A summary of the evidence from migration studies supports the following hypotheses:

1 that breast cancer risk is primarily determined by environmental and not genetic factors (although genetic traits have been confirmed for about 5% of all racial groups)
2 that early migration is associated with increased nutrition during childhood and the peripubertal period, which is associated with an early menarche, which in turn is associated with increased breast cancer risk
3 that migration is associated with increased weight during adult life, particularly during the postmenopausal years, which in turn is associated with a modest increase in risk of breast cancer.

Deferral of first pregnancy and changes in alcohol consumption by migrants may also influence their risk of breast cancer.

TABLE 4.1 Premenopausal breast cancer mortality among female migrants to Australia from Italy and Greece from 1966 to 1994: a comparison between those who migrated before and after the age of 20 years
This information suggests that changes in the environment in the new host country affect young people to nearly double the extent of older people. The relative risk between those who migrated before the age of 20 years compared with those who migrated after the age of 20 years is approximately double for both Italian and Greek migrants. It is likely that it is the increased consumption of rich food in the host country that increases both growth and maturity in young migrants, which in turn increases subsequent breast cancer risk. Other plausible explanations are changes in fertility patterns, such as deferral of first pregnancy, and changes in alcohol consumption.

		Relative risk
ITALY	Migrated < age 20 years	1.6
	Migrated > age 20 years	1.0
GREECE	Migrated < age 20 years	2.2
	Migrated > age 20 years	1.0

Source: Australian Bureau of Statistics, unpublished data.

is there proof of the effects of diet?

Because of the observations outlined in the previous chapter—that people who consume diets rich in energy, fats and proteins, such as residents of the US and the UK, have much higher rates of breast cancer than people from predominantly cereal-eating countries such as China and Japan—there has been an intense scientific effort aimed at proving a link between diet (in particular, fats) and breast cancer. This effort has turned out to be both difficult and disappointing.

In recent years we have become accustomed to reading about the latest medical discovery, proving a relationship between our diet and our diseases. It seems that each week a new relationship is uncovered: a high-salt diet leads to high blood pressure and an increased risk of heart disease; too little fibre increases chances of cancer of the colon; too much food altogether and you are more likely to develop diabetes. Perhaps the most popular discovery was that drinking one or two glasses of red wine each day lowers the risk of heart disease—discovered when it was noticed that the French, who have a relatively high-fat diet, don't seem to be dying of heart attacks as a result, and all because they like wine (particularly red wine) with their cheese. These discoveries are usually embraced by the public. In a world where things all too often seem out of our control, learning about how the food we eat can affect our bodies is almost always considered a positive step. If we control little else, we can at least decide what to eat.

Scientific conclusions explained

To date, the consumption of foods such as meat, fruit and vegetables has not been shown to have much impact on breast cancer.

First, it is important to understand why, despite innumerable tests, there are so many 'ifs, buts and maybes'—as well as so many approximations—in the reduced, or increased, risk percentages when discussing the connection between the consumption of certain foods and the risk of breast cancer.

Often the best conclusion anyone can come to after these long and expensive studies is that the association between diet and breast cancer may or may not be true, and may or may not be **causal**.

The term 'causal' is common in scientific writing. It refers to a factor being the actual cause of a disease as distinct from being merely associated with the disease. Often a factor that is thought to be causal—where it actually affects the risk of getting the disease—turns out to be an association.

This is well illustrated by the 'bra theory'. Researchers such as the American husband and wife team, Sydney Singer and Soma Grismaijer, have noted that in countries where the wearing of bras is common, such as the US and Europe, breast cancer rates are high; and as soon as women in a developing country such as Fiji start wearing bras, breast cancer rates rise. They speculate that the bra constricts the lymphatic drainage system and stops the clearance of toxic substances, which may lead to an elevated risk of breast cancer. For proof they point to the furrows in the skin readily seen when the bra is removed before going to bed. Singer and Grismaijer have published a book outlining their observations and theories,[1] but do not appear to have had their work accepted in the scientific literature.

---

a factor that is **causal** helps to cause the disease

However, their observations are accurate: women in the US and Europe wear bras and also have high rates of breast cancer, and the occurrence of breast cancer in Fijian women is rising. Although these associations are not due to chance, neither are they causal. The probable real association is that economic expansion has led to the consumption of increasingly rich food by Fijian women, as well as the purchasing and wearing of bras, and it is the food not the bra that is the cause of increased breast cancer in Fiji. Wearing a bra almost certainly does not influence the risk of breast cancer, and is not a causal factor. The studies by Singer and Grismaijer did not follow established scientific methods and hence arrived at misleading results.

Often, however, it has been found impossible to determine absolutely whether a link between food and breast cancer is causal or just associated. The difficulty is that we live in a society where experimenting with animals is highly controversial and scientific studies on humans are often practically impossible. For example, it is obviously impractical to consider recruiting a large number of children and giving them an experimental diet for 50 years and then comparing their experience of breast cancer with that of another group fed a different diet, also for 50 years. The only realistic way such a study can be conducted is with volunteer groups of women, such as the participants in *The Nurses Health Study*, and among women who have developed breast cancer. Such studies are referred to as 'prospective studies' and 'case-control studies' respectively.

Prospective studies offer more accurate results than case-control studies. This is largely because case-control studies, where the women have already developed breast cancer, can be biased by the selection of the **cases** and the controls, and by the women under study unconsciously giving answers aimed at pleasing the researchers. We need to consider what is meant by **controls**. An essential principle of scientific research is to compare one group of

---

prospective study research method that looks at the characteristics of people before they develop a disease

cases the experimental group

controls the comparison group

subjects, whether humans or animals, with another group. In this way, the effect of a medicine or vaccine given to one group can be measured by comparison with the other 'control' group. The difficulty lies in ensuring that the experimental group and the control group are as equal as possible in all ways except for the medicine or vaccine. This is much easier said than done; scientists are human too and may unconsciously bias their results to the expected outcome—that is, that the medicine or vaccine works. Also, the participants in such studies may forget their past experiences, or colour their memories, or seek to give 'appropriate' answers to questions in order to please the researchers. Hence we see the value of prospective studies where the outcome is not known at the beginning of the study.

But there are problems with both types of studies. When researching possible links between food and cancer, the most difficult problem is to measure accurately the food consumption of the participants, in both prospective and case-control studies. It is not practical to have an independent observer watching and recording the details of food eaten by each subject, 24 hours each day, in a study that may include more than 100 000 participants. Also, the mere presence of an observer is known to bias behaviour. For these reasons dietary histories, as distinct from first-hand observations, are made for each participant. This can be done simply by asking subjects to recall their food consumption for the previous 24 hours or to keep a detailed diary of the food they eat. Both methods give reasonable results but are not completely reliable.

Additional problems arise with respect to the nature of the population being studied. For example, food consumption, particularly of fat, is much higher in the US than in Japan. As an indication of the difference, the lowest consumption levels of fats by individuals in many American studies is greater than the highest consumption levels of fat by individuals in Japan. Thus it is difficult to compare the results of studies between countries.

This problem is demonstrated by studies of the possible protective effect of vitamins against breast cancer. No protective effect (or only a small protective effect for vitamin A) of vitamins A and C has been shown in US-based studies[2] which contrasts with China-based and Japan-based studies.[3-8] These differences may well be due to the influence of markedly different fat consumption levels between the two populations.

Despite the problems, these two types of studies are the best we have available. The following is an overview of what we now know and, in some cases, what we suspect.

Fat

Fat and calories (energy) are closely correlated in the diet. High consumption of fats is almost always associated with high consumption of total energy. This is because fats in general, and animal-sourced fats in particular, are concentrated sources of energy. For this reason, studies that aim to observe the influence of fats are difficult to interpret as the influence may be due to either the fats or the energy.

Early interest in a possible association between consumption of fats and breast cancer came from Albert Tannenbaum, who conducted pioneering studies on mice in Chicago during the 1940s.[9,10] He showed convincingly that diets high in fat increased the occurrence of **mammary tumours** in mice.

It was this work that stimulated the population studies by Armstrong and Doll that were discussed earlier.[11] With both the animal and population studies suggesting that high consumption of fat was the breast cancer culprit, hopes were high, and case-control research studies aimed at finally proving the link were initiated in many countries during the 1970s and 1980s. These countries included the US, Argentina, Australia, China, Canada, Greece, Israel and Italy.

---

mammary tumour a tumour in the breast

Geoffrey Howe, of the National Cancer Institute in Toronto, reviewed 12 of these studies in 1990 and concluded that in relation to postmenopausal cancer (generally affecting women from their mid-forties onwards), those who had a diet high in fats, particularly animal fats, were increasing their risk of breast cancer.[12] High concentrations of animal fats are found in all meats, particularly red meat, in butter and in products that use butter, such as biscuits, pastries and cakes. By comparing women in a particular population (e.g. a suburb), it was determined that those women with a high consumption of saturated (mainly animal) fats had a 50% greater risk than those women with a low consumption.[12]

This information spread rapidly and was probably an influential force in the decision to begin breast cancer prevention trials aimed at reducing the consumption of fat in American women. To test the theory, groups of women were placed on low-fat diets, over an extended period of time, to determine whether their risk of breast cancer dropped. The expected results were not confirmed by the slowly emerging prospective studies.[13]

By definition, prospective trials are slow and, because of the intensive effort involved, very expensive. A good prospective trial can take 20 or even 40 years (as in the case of smoking and the British doctors' study) to complete. The key prospective studies looking at a possible fat and breast cancer link have been uniformly negative.[13] Contrary to the work of Geoffrey Howe, they show no connection between fat and breast cancer risk. In addition, they have not shown that breast cancer had any link with the consumption of total energy.

There is a problem in all these studies. They all measure the food consumption of adults—they do not measure food consumption in children and teenagers. This was to prove to be a major omission and a much needed clue to the elusive origins of breast cancer.

Fruits, vegetables and vitamins

Vitamin A has two vital roles to play. The first is a key role in vision. Deficiency of vitamin A occurs in many developing countries where it is commonly associated with partial or full loss of vision, particularly in children. Its second role is relevant to breast cancer: vitamin A is an important regulator of cell multiplication and specialisation and may influence the prevention of malignant change in cells. The cells in the body are continually replacing themselves. For some types of cells this replacement is quick, as in the case of blood cells, for others it is slow, as for bone and brain cells. This replacement requires cells to divide and multiply and during this process mistakes can be made and the cells can become cancerous. Specialisation of cells occurs as the body matures. The relevant example are breast cells, which specialise during pregnancy so they can produce milk for the baby.

Common dietary sources of vitamin A in developed countries are dairy products such as milk, cheese, butter and icecream, plus products made from animal livers, and fish such as herring, tuna and sardines. Common food sources of substances known as carotenoids, which are converted by the body into vitamin A, are coloured fruits and vegetables such as carrots, corn, tomatoes, papaya, oranges and spinach.

Some other vitamins and nutrients, known as **antioxidants**, may also be associated with the protection of the genetic material in cells and ensure safe regulated cell multiplication.

Hence the interest in these substances.

Theoretically, it is likely that vitamin A would reduce the risk of breast cancer. Most, but not all, prospective and case-control studies suggest there is a protective effect of about 20–30% from the consumption of vegetables and fruits containing vitamin A.[12,14-16] Results from prospective studies of vitamin C, which is also contained in fruits and vegetables, and which is an antioxidant and again, theoretically, should provide some protection, are inconsistent

---

antioxidants agents, such as vitamins, that inhibit oxidation. An example of oxidation is the deterioration of fats (rancidity) when exposed to the oxygen in the air

and no conclusions can be made.[14,15] Deficiency of vitamin C leads to the historical disease of scurvy.

Although vitamin E is an antioxidant and is required for growth, particularly of reproductive tissues, various studies have not shown that it has any protective effects.[14,15] Vitamin E is contained in grains, nuts, sunflower seeds and corn.

The possible protection offered by vitamins (almost solely confined to vitamin A) leads to the question of whether supplements such as vitamin pills can reduce breast cancer risk? It has been found that, unless you have a very low intake of vitamin A (as a result of not consuming enough fruit and vegetables), there are no benefits in taking vitamin supplements as protection against breast cancer.[14,15] However, fruit and vegetables are effective in reducing cancers of the colon and lung and, in the Western world, where it is difficult to increase people's consumption of fruit and vegetables, vitamin supplements can be generally beneficial.

But people do not naturally eat vitamins. We eat fruit and vegetables. It may be that the influence of eating an apple is different from the influence of eating a single vitamin in the form of a vitamin pill. There is no strong evidence that this notion is accurate.

Kristi Steinmetz and John Potter, who work in the World Cancer Research Fund in London, have recently reviewed over 200 research studies in both humans and animals which seek an answer to the question: 'Does consumption of fruit and vegetables reduce the risk of cancer?' The evidence is strong and clear that there is a protective effect of about 50% from greater consumption of fruit and vegetables for cancers of the stomach, oesophagus, lung, endometrium (lining of the womb), pancreas (the gland in the abdomen that produces insulin) and the colon.

The evidence that increased consumption of fruit and vegetables protects against breast cancer is not as strong, but 75% of studies suggest there is some protective effect.

While virtually all types of fruit and vegetables offer some protection, raw vegetables are particularly effective.[17]

Dietary fibre

At one stage it was thought that diets high in fibre might offer protection against breast cancer because fibre may reduce the absorption of oestrogens. This was initially confirmed in an animal experiment[18] but has not been shown to be the case in any major studies in humans.[19]

Soy and phytoestrogens

Soy products, such as tofu, contain plant oestrogens (hence the name **phytoestrogens**—'phyto' means plant in ancient Greek) and have been suggested as one of the factors responsible for the low rate of breast cancer in high tofu-consuming Chinese populations.[20]

This is an interesting possibility but is not supported by the largest study so far into diet and breast cancer in China.[21] On the other hand, a recent Australian study which measured the urinary excretion of plant oestrogens as an indication of consumption levels showed that they possibly did provide some protection.[22] This was a small study and so the findings must be treated with caution. Obviously, much more work is needed on this issue before policies of prevention can be developed.

However, many women have turned to 'natural' remedies and, because of concern about the possible risk of breast cancer associated with hormone replacement therapy, there is increased use of products and food that contain phytoestrogens at the age of menopause. So, although there is no strong evidence to support the use of phytoestrogens to prevent breast cancer, some background information is of interest.

Phytoestrogens are found in many natural foods. These foods include whole grains such as wheat, barley, rice bran and oat bran, legumes such as beans and peas, vegetables such as carrots, alfalfa,

phytoestrogens oestrogens sourced from plants

onions and corn, fruits such as apples, pears, cherries and stone fruits, soy beans, soyflour, soy milk and other soy products and, in addition, garlic, olive oil and sunflower seeds. So a broadly based diet containing fruit and vegetables will almost certainly contain phytoestrogens.

Phytoestrogens are complex chemicals and contain both oestrogens and anti-oestrogens at the same time. The anti-oestrogen effect should theoretically reduce breast cancer and, indeed, phytoestrogens have been shown to reduce cancer activity in experimental animals. One study conducted in Singapore is compatible with the hypothesis, but does not prove, that diets high in phytoestrogens (in this case, soy foods) reduce breast cancer by about 30% in premenopausal women.[23]

The effects of phytoestrogens on the foetus of experimental mice have recently been reported. Contrary to expectations, phytoestrogens appear to act as oestrogen in the uterus and may increase the risk of breast cancer in female mouse offspring.[23a]

Soy foods have been used with safety for millennia in China and elsewhere and their use can be encouraged, but expectations with respect to breast cancer prevention must be treated with caution.

Olive oil

The hypothesis that fat intake increases the risk of breast cancer (which was discussed earlier and does not appear to be true in the case of adults) has so dominated the scientific debate that little consideration has been given to the possibility that some forms of fat may actually reduce breast cancer.

Olive oil is one such fat. There are only four studies available that examine this issue, two from Spain, one from Greece and one from Italy. All four are case-control studies and so not totally reliable, but they do indicate a modest (approximately 25%) benefit in reducing the risk of breast cancer by the consumption of olive oil.[24-27] This is supported by studies in animals. The underlying chemistry, which would explain why this is the case, is poorly understood.

The key characteristic of olive oil is that it is a major source of monounsaturated fats. Monounsaturated fats are also found in dairy, meat and margarine products. A recent small but reliable prospective study in Sweden has shown that consumption of monounsaturated fats may reduce breast cancer by up to 50%.[28] These research findings have a number of implications. The first is that it is the monounsaturated fats that offer the protection from breast cancer and not the olive oil. However, olive oil is one of the highest sources of monounsaturated fats available. Second, it is not known at which age the consumption of monounsaturated fats has the most influence. This influence of monounsaturated fats is in contrast to polyunsaturated fats, which are high in vegetable margarines and cereals, and which were found in the Swedish study to be associated with about a 20% increase in risk of breast cancer. There was no association between saturated fats and breast cancer. Saturated fats are high in meat and dairy products and are strongly associated with increased coronary heart disease.

Despite the complex nature of these different types of fat, attention has to be given to the possibility that there are many different types of fat and they have differing influences. Therefore it is helpful to offer some explanation about fats.

There is no accepted definition of the word 'fat' although most of us know what fat is! However, nutritionists distinguish between 'visible' and 'invisible' fats. Visible fats include the fat on meat, and in butter, margarines and cooking oils. Invisible fats are hidden during cooking and there may be quite high levels of fats in cakes, biscuits, potato chips and crisps and a wide range of processed meats and sausages. Also, these fats vary widely in chemical composition and in their effect on the body chemistry and ultimately on disease processes.

Fat is composed of three basic chemicals: carbon, hydrogen and oxygen. In simple terms, a fat is classified as saturated, monounsaturated or polyunsaturated depending on the combination of the three basic chemicals in it. There are many different types of fats within each of these three main groups. *Saturated fats*, which are concentrated in dairy products and meats from domesticated animals, are well known because their consumption is associated with high levels of coronary artery disease (a condition associated with the formation of fatty deposits in the walls of the arteries, ultimately leading to blockage of the arteries). The consumption of *monounsaturated* and *polyunsaturated fats*, which are concentrated in olives and oil-bearing plants such as soybeans and sunflowers, have a much lower influence on atherosclerotic (thickening of the arteries) processes.

There is strong consistent evidence from experimental studies on rats and mice that diets high in monounsaturated fats have a protective effect against mammary tumours. In contrast, diets high in polyunsaturated fats increase the risk of mammary tumours. Experiments on pregnant rats have shown that diets high in polyunsaturated fats increase mammary tumours in female offspring.

Given the limited information available, in most circumstances it would be imprudent to make any recommendations. However, the consumption of monounsaturated fats from olive oil has been associated with reduction in risk of coronary heart disease; therefore, it is safe to suggest, despite the incomplete evidence, that consumption of olive oil and other sources of monounsaturated fats—instead of dairy products, fried 'fast foods' and fatty meats—is a reasonable approach aimed at some reduction in risk of breast cancer.

Western diets are unsafely high in most forms of fat. Fat does contain many essential nutrients, but it has long been known that radical reductions in total fat consumption are very safe. The most obvious example of the safety and desirability of radical reduction in fats in the diet is the uniquely high health status of Japanese men and women, who consume 20% less total fat than their Western counterparts.

Selenium

Selenium is a chemical found in soils from where it enters the food chain through cereals, fruits and vegetables. The concentrations in soils vary from area to area. It is a **micronutrient** (a component of food that is present in tiny but often essential amounts—iodine is a good example: low iodine leads to brain damage in infants) and associated with antioxidant activities. Antioxidants are involved with the control of cell multiplication and hence are relevant to cancerous cell multiplication.

Experiments in animals consistently show that selenium offers protection against a wide range of cancers. Because the intake of selenium varies so greatly among humans, depending on the selenium content of soils, it has not been possible to assess intake in dietary surveys. Surprisingly enough, the most accurate way of measuring selenium intake is by examining toenail clippings, rather than blood or other body fluids. Many studies have been conducted into the relationship between selenium and breast cancer where the level of selenium intake has been ascertained via the toenail. These studies do not confirm any influence of selenium on breast cancer risk.[29]

Coffee and tea

Even coffee has been a suspect as a risk for breast cancer. Many studies have examined this possibility but no associations have been observed.[30]

There have been many reports, based on experiments with animals, that drinking tea may lower the risk of cancer in general. These findings are compatible with the casual observation that breast cancer and some other cancers are lower in Japan than in Western countries and, as the drinking of green tea is a common custom in Japan, there might be a link. Sadly, there appears to be no scientific support for these theories. Very sound studies conducted in the US and Holland have clearly shown there is no protection against breast cancer by

---

micronutrients are present in food in tiny but often essential amounts

drinking even large quantities of black tea.[31,32] Similar studies in Japan have found no protection from drinking green tea.[33] Green tea may offer some protection against cancer of the colon but, again, additional studies are required.

Dairy products

There is substantial, but not conclusive, evidence that consumption of dairy products may be associated with increased risk of breast cancer. It is obviously important to offer an outline of this evidence because of the adverse implications to both women and the dairy industry. There are more than a dozen studies indicating a possible association between dairy product consumption and breast cancer risk. This evidence has been recently reviewed by Outwater and colleagues from Princeton University.[34] Their evidence shows that, if there is such an association, it is cheese and whole milk that offer the most adverse influences. However, it must be stated that there are four studies that are inconclusive or show no risk from dairy product consumption.

If there is such an association, there are several possible mechanisms apart from the influence of dietary fat content. One is the possible influence of chemicals present in dairy products, called insulin-like growth factors; these are normal components of the body and are necessary for normal growth, but when present in excess may be associated with malignant disease. Another possibility is that milk may function as transport for cancer-producing chemicals. This suggestion is based on an experience in Israel where it was found that cow growth hormones, given to promote milk production, may have been responsible for an increase followed by a decline in breast cancer in Israeli women. The decline followed the removal of these growth hormone contaminants from cows and their milk.[35,36]

Although many more studies are required it is at least possible that consumption of dairy products is associated with possible risk of breast cancer.

Diet during adolescence

There has been increased interest in the possible influence of diet during adolescence on breast cancer risk. This interest is based on three things: the reduced risk of breast cancer among women whose diet was restricted in adolescence during World War II; the link between early age at menarche and increased risk of breast cancer; and the observation that the earlier the age of achieving maximum height the greater the risk of subsequent breast cancer.[37-39]

A recent large study among adolescent females in the United States has considered this issue. They have not been able to show any influence of diet during adolescence on the risk of early onset breast cancer. However, this finding does not exclude the influence of diet on preadolescent children, particularly with respect to the influences of diet on the age at menarche.[40]

Despite enormous and expensive studies in many parts of the world, the hypothesis that fat could be a major risk factor for breast cancer appears to have been more often refuted than supported. This is very discouraging, because the fat/breast cancer hypothesis had appeared to be the most promising. But were the studies based on an incorrect or incomplete hypothesis? The answer to this question is probably yes and no, because of the concentration of studies into diets consumed during adult life, not during early life.

However, many believe that the central hypothesis—that fats or high-energy foods are related to breast cancer—is still valid, despite the evidence that has been presented to the contrary. So we are left with a contradictory message: on the one hand there is circumstantial evidence of a connection between consumption of fats, energy and breast cancer risk; on the other hand there is direct evidence to refute this!

Despite the evidence to the contrary, there is a reason for the seemingly 'wishful' belief that fats and other high-energy foods and, probably, proteins may well be highly influential in the development of breast cancer. Tannenbaum and his mice may have unintentionally misled a generation of researchers. Such was his fame in this field of research that, when he commented that age was not a factor in the increased risk of breast cancer in fat-fed mice, it became an accepted fact.

However, after a careful review of Tannenbaum's data,[9,10] (which can still be found in any substantial biomedical library 50 years after it was first published), there is evidence to show that the fats he fed to young mice had a greater influence on mouse breast cancer risk than the same fats fed to older mice. In a paper published in 1942 Tannenbaum stated 'it is obviously unnecessary that calorie restriction be instituted at a very early age in order that breast tumour formation be inhibited'.[9]

But Tannenbaum's statement is not in accord with his results. The results of his study on calorie restriction in mice show that no mice placed on a calorie-restricted diet at 10 weeks of age developed mammary tumours at 20 months of age, compared with the controls who were fed standard diets and who developed many mammary tumours.[9]

Similarly, in another experiment[10] on the effects of a high-fat diet in mice, Tannenbaum showed that mice placed on a high-fat diet at 18–32 weeks of age had twice the number of spontaneous mammary tumours than mice placed on identical diets at 32–48 weeks of age. Mice aged 18–32 weeks of age can be regarded as pubertal, those 32–48 weeks of age as postpubertal.

Experiments in recent years have confirmed these conclusions. With almost no exception, the dozens of case-control and prospective studies that have been conducted on human adults have assumed that the only diet under the 'causal' question is the adult diet. What has not been considered is that humans may be sensitive to the influence of fat and energy intake only at 'sensitive' times in their lives, at an age where the causal effects of diet have not been previously considered—that is, until the completion of a very recent and very important study.[41]

Way back in the 1930s, Lord Boyd Orr studied and recorded the diet and health status of families and their children in the United Kingdom. Over 60 years later these children were identified as adults and their health status was again reviewed. Of course, many had died but the causes of their deaths could be identified. It was found that those who had a higher consumption of energy as children subsequently had higher death rates from all cancers as both male and female adults, except for those cancers related to tobacco smoking. The findings included breast cancer, for which there was an approximate increase of about 10% among those adults who had consumed higher-energy diets as children. This confirms, in humans, Tannenbaum's early studies in animals.

In view of the obvious importance of these observations to the risk of breast cancer these issues are explored in detail later in the book.

 Thus far, diet has offered only modest clues. These are:

- Vitamin A and olive oil both probably offer some protection, say 25% reduction in risk.
- Experience from China, where olive oil is not a normal part of the diet, suggests that vitamin A and olive oil appear to act independently.
- It may be that phytoestrogens (plant-sourced oestrogens) offer some protection—but sound evidence is not yet available.
- Fats consumed in adult life do not pose a major breast cancer risk (although they may cause excess weight in postmenopausal women).
- A range of nutrients and foods, including vitamin C, selenium, fibre, soy and coffee, are not relevant.

Walter Willett—workaholic

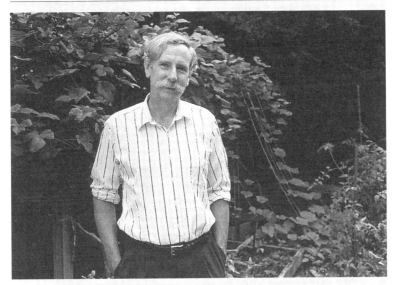

Based at the School of Public Health at Harvard University, Walter Willett, together with colleagues, has been responsible for the enormous US *Nurses Health Study* which has provided many new insights into the causes of breast cancer.

WALTER WILLETT is one of those absolutely brilliant, compulsive, workaholic researchers found on every United States university campus. Browsing through the references at the end of this book you will see his name appearing on a regular basis. He publishes a scientific paper at the rate of about one per week. By way of comparison, for most of us, one paper per year is okay. The assumption that there is no value in volume does not apply to Walter, whose work is of great importance because of his role in *The Nurses Health Study*, to which he has contributed on a continuing basis for over 20 years.

His specialty is nutrition and epidemiology.

Walter is inclined to some dogmatism and is therefore prone to making pronouncements without qualification. In the epidemiologic field, this is considered to be a dangerous activity and it has frequently caused the wrath of the food industry to fall on Walter.

His dogmatism is exactly what is needed in this field. While, clearly, it would be misleading if all epidemiologists offered such firm opinions, Walter's forthright pronouncements have generally stood the test of time. These include his support for the consumption of monounsaturated fats, found in olive oil and fish, as a protection against coronary heart disease and his disdain for the saturated fats from dairy and meat products that increase heart disease.

Walter eats data for breakfast. He sits in a modest, hopelessly cluttered office in the back of the Harvard School of Public Health, surrounded by papers and computers. To visitors, the scene is one of chaos, but to Walter every piece of paper has its place and will eventually contribute to a new scientific publication.

Like many physicians who have developed an interest in the priority of prevention over treatment of disease, Walter spent a period working in a developing country— in his case, Tanzania. In such countries the importance of prevention is obvious in contrast to technically developed societies where the brilliance of technology tends to obscure the equal need for prevention. Walter has sought to put the results of his many studies into practice by his vigorous advocacy of a healthy diet and lifestyle. This combination of scientific rigour and public advocacy has made Walter Willett a model and hero to a generation of epidemiologists.

6

physical factors and social class

Physical factors

To the casual observer, possible links between breast cancer and height, weight, obesity and whether a female has big or little breasts seems obscure. However, these issues have been matters of intense research interest, mainly because weight and breast size are associated with dietary patterns—a topic that has dominated the search for the key to breast cancer prevention.

Weight for height

Research findings with respect to weight are almost exactly the opposite of the researchers' expectations. Study after study has consistently found that excess weight in premenopausal women may actually reduce the risk of breast cancer by 10–20%—or, at the very least, not increase the risk as expected.[1-3]

The exception may be found in the very few studies conducted among populations with low breast cancer risk, such as Asia, where all show an increased risk of breast cancer among women who are overweight.[4,5] However, in these studies no distinction has been made between premenopausal and postmenopausal women.

From an international perspective, women from economically developing countries who are tall and heavy for height are at greater risk of breast cancer than short, light women.[6] Studies from economically developed countries, particularly the US, offer a confused picture. Some studies, such as *The Nurses Health Study*, have shown no substantial link between breast cancer and excess weight in postmenopausal women.[7] This study also showed a reduction in risk among premenopausal women who were overweight. This is in contrast to other more recent studies of US and Dutch women which have shown that breast cancer risk is greater among tall and obese postmenopausal women.[1,8] In addition, short black US women are at less risk than their tall black counterparts.[9]

This is, of course, extremely confusing and appears to run counter to the firm evidence that fat consumption in adult women has no impact on breast cancer risk.

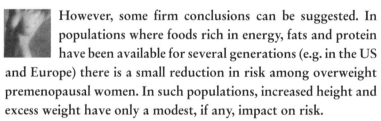 **However, some firm conclusions can be suggested. In populations where foods rich in energy, fats and protein have been available for several generations (e.g. in the US and Europe) there is a small reduction in risk among overweight premenopausal women. In such populations, increased height and excess weight have only a modest, if any, impact on risk.**

However, in populations where 'rich' diets are not universally available, such as in China, tall, overweight women (who presumably have access to richer diets than other Chinese women) are at double the risk of postmenopausal breast cancer.[4]

A fascinating insight into this issue has been provided by a recent study into the experience of Asian-American women, aged 20–55 years, living in San Francisco, Los Angeles and Hawaii.[8] It was found that overweight women in their fifties (postmenopausal) had twice the risk of breast cancer compared with thinner women of the same age. Women who had gained more than 4 kilos (about 9 pounds) during the previous decade of their lives experienced an even greater increase in the risk of breast cancer (up to three times the risk) compared with women who had no weight change. An increase in weight of 4 kilos over a 10 year period does not seem much to a Western woman, but even such a modest gain appears to offer an adverse influence. The term being used to describe this phenomenon is 'late stage promotion'.

The formal conclusion is that excess weight may act as a late stage promoter of breast cancer.

By the end of 1997 a possible explanation had emerged for the contradictory observation that obese premenopausal women were at reduced risk and obese postmenopausal women at increased risk of breast cancer. The explanation is based on three separate studies, which showed:

1   that obesity in premenopausal women reduces the number of ovulations and hence hormone levels[10]

2   rapid weight gain (i.e. over about five years) increases hormone levels in postmenopausal women[8] and

3   US nurses who were postmenopausal and overweight, and who had never used hormone replacement therapy, had a higher risk of breast cancer than their counterparts who used hormone replacement therapy.[11] The implication of this third observation is that excess fat tissues produce hormones at levels above those from hormone replacement therapy.

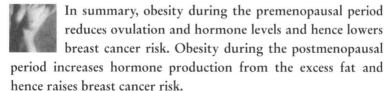

In summary, obesity during the premenopausal period reduces ovulation and hormone levels and hence lowers breast cancer risk. Obesity during the postmenopausal period increases hormone production from the excess fat and hence raises breast cancer risk.

An obvious prevention measure for all women, especially those of postmenopausal age, is to avoid obesity and in particular rapid weight gain.

Height

Adult height is determined by a range of factors including genetics, experiences of infections and, above all, diet. Americans and Australians are currently on average about 15 centimetres (6 inches) taller than their great-grandparents were at the turn of the century. Young Japanese now tower over their parents. Afro-Americans are huge, even when compared with modern Nigerians and other West Africans. Diet is the dominant factor in this 'growth' phenomenon.

Because there is almost no increase in height after 20 years of age, height is a good indicator of nutritional experience during childhood and adolescence. For this reason researchers have looked for links between height and breast cancer, with height as a surrogate measure of nutrition during the period of growth. However, the argument or observation is circular as nutrition stimulates growth and growth itself appears to be a risk factor for breast cancer.

Some of these studies have involved vast numbers of women. For example, Steinar Tretli working from Oslo in Norway has studied the risk of breast cancer in more than 500 000 women for nearly 20 years.[12] He has found a weak but consistently positive association between height and increased risk of breast cancer.

The results of these studies provide evidence that height is modestly associated with increased risk of breast cancer and, conversely, that short stature decreases risk.[13] This latter observation has been confirmed in US black women where shortness was proven to reduce the risk by half.[9]

In late 1997 a new insight about height emerged from the United States. It appears that the earlier the age a female reaches her maximum height, the greater the risk of breast cancer.[14] For example, if a female grows to 5 feet 9 inches (about 175 centimetres) by age 15 years there is about a 30% increase in risk compared with a female who reaches the same height at 18 years. This early attainment of maximum height correlates with early menarche—that is, girls who have early menarche also attain maximum height at an early age.

Elizabeth Sutherland fitted this profile. She grew early and she grew taller than her parents. Presumably this was because she had access to an even richer diet than her parents. It is now known that early growth and tall height increase risk of breast cancer.

 So, height has provided a substantial clue. Height is associated with growth, growth is associated with nutrition, nutrition is associated with age at menarche. The factors are interrelated and it may be that they are all influences on breast cancer risk.

Large breasts

On the international scale, American, Australian and European women have big breasts. They are also at higher risk of breast cancer than their small-chested counterparts. Chinese, Japanese and Korean women, who have small breasts, have a lower risk of breast cancer. There is obviously an association between breast size and breast cancer, but this association is probably not causal.

We have already spoken about the meaning of the word 'causal'. The term is used in research papers to distinguish between possible risk factors that *contribute to the cause of a disease*, and those factors that are *associated* with the disease but do not contribute to the cause. For example, rising incomes are associated with increased risk of coronary heart disease, but such incomes are not causal. Rising incomes allow the consumption of fatty foods to be increased; it is the fatty foods that are causal for coronary heart disease, not the incomes.

Knowledge about breast size of populations is a delicate issue, but size can be broadly assessed from the purchasing patterns of bras. Because bras are adopted when economies develop, an accurate record of bra purchases, and breast sizes, can be gained only from

Western countries and from the city dweller in countries such as China and Korea. It is obvious that Western women have much larger busts than Asian women, but this does not imply that large breasts are a factor in breast cancer risk. The lack of an independent causal association between breast size and breast cancer has recently been confirmed by a Dutch research team led by David Beijerinck.[15]

Breast structure

When breast tissues are examined by X-ray, shadows or patterns known as **parenchyma** can be seen. When these parenchyma are dense, it can be an early signal that the patient has an increased risk of breast cancer. This finding was first observed in 1960 by Ingleby and Gershon-Cohen and led to the development of X-ray mammography which has allowed early breast cancer to be detected and treated.[16]

Helpful though these observations proved to be in early detection, they give no additional clues to the cause of breast cancer.

Breast augmentation and cancer

The popularity of body building, silicon implants, and boosting the size of the bosom with injections offers proof of the importance of breasts to both men and women. It has been estimated that since the 1960s, in the US alone, more than two million women have augmented their breasts with silicon implants.

But are silicon implants safe?

There has been concern about the safety of silicon implants for some time. This concern came to a head when several recipients became seriously ill, apparently because of reactions to leaks of silicon from its capsule inside the breast. Dow Corning, the Michigan-based manufacturer of breast implants, was severely criticised for marketing the product before appropriate safety checks were conducted. In

---

parenchyma shadows or patterns in the breast

January 1992, the US Food and Drug Administration called for a moratorium on the use of breast augmentation devices until detailed safety checks were carried out.

The initial concerns were based on single-case reports. While such reports can be very helpful, they can also be quite misleading; systematic research has often demonstrated the cause of a problem to be quite different from that hypothesised by single-case reports. With respect to silicon implants the case reports were subsequently shown to be misleading. Reliable studies from Minnesota did not reveal any problems with silicon implants.[17] Additional, more detailed, studies from the US and Sweden have confirmed these early conclusions that there does not appear to be any connection between silicon breast implants and a range of diseases, particularly connective tissue diseases such as rheumatoid arthritis and inflammation of the muscles and fibrous tissues.[18–21]

However, there is some evidence that silicon implants may be associated with a small increase in risk of several rare cancers including sarcoma (cancer of the connective tissues), multiple myeloma and other cancers of the blood-forming cells. These risks appear to be low, but further studies are needed before complete safety can be guaranteed.

With respect to breast cancer there is a problem associated with the reduced visibility of the breast tissue during mammography following implants, but of course this has no bearing on the issue of any possible relationship between silicon and increased risk of cancer.

Breast cancer and social class

During the 1970s I was responsible for organising and managing the public health services of northern Sydney, Australia, on behalf of some one million citizens. An essential part of the planning was to review the patterns of disease among the various social groups that lived in the city. Breast cancer was an obvious problem for two reasons: first, it was a serious, common and increasing problem; second, it was the only disease that was more common in the wealthier parts of the population. While poor people may not regard this as a problem, the observation is of considerable interest because breast cancer is one of the few causes of death that are more common in rich people.

We blamed the poor quality of the data for this observation, but the pattern persisted each year. I was to learn that what we were experiencing was a pattern that had been found in many countries over many years, even in 'classless' communist China. The differences were substantial, at about 10–20% greater risk of breast cancer for top female income earners as compared with those with the lowest incomes.

The behaviour and health of people varies dramatically according to socioeconomic status, that is, social class. This is the reason for developing and recording information that can measure social class reasonably accurately. One of the most obvious examples of class-related behaviour is voting patterns. High-income earners tend to vote for conservative political parties such as the Republicans in the US, and the Conservatives in the UK, while low-income earners mostly support union-based left-wing political parties such as the Labo(u)r parties in Australia and the UK.

In economically developed countries, death rates for almost all medical conditions, except breast cancer, tend to be higher among low-income, low socioeconomic status people.[22] For example, death rates among process workers due to coronary heart disease, lung cancer and even traffic accidents are double those of professional and technical workers. The reasons for these differences are complex but are usually attributed to 'lifestyle' factors, which are shaped by the education and culture of the social group. It is not that socioeconomic status itself is a risk factor, but it gives a fairly accurate indication of health-related patterns and risks, such as smoking and eating habits, as well as behaviour trends, within a social and economic grouping.

Casual observation of the people around you will readily confirm these findings. Take a discreet look at the shopping trolleys of working and professional class people as they queue at the supermarket checkout. Working class shopping patterns tend to include bulk cigarettes, fatty mince meats and lots of biscuits and coke. In contrast, professional class shoppers tend to buy whole grain bread, lean meat and plenty of vegetables and fruit. Professional and technical citizens walk and jog; they tend to be slim and few smoke. They live a long time. Process workers are more likely to be overweight smokers who rarely exercise. They are less concerned about being considered 'responsible drivers' and, as a result, they are involved in more car accidents. Working class people tend to become seriously ill at an earlier age and will often die in their sixties.

However, these patterns do not apply to breast cancer (see Table 6.1).

Table 6.1 Breast cancer risk between lowest and highest social group from eight countries; socioeconomic status measured by education and occupation
The differences in breast cancer incidence and mortality rates are greatest where there is a wide range of socioeconomic status in the same population. The differences decline as socioeconomic inequalities in a particular population decline. This is illustrated by the high relative risk of breast cancer among educated as compared with uneducated women in China, an intermediate relative risk in Italy, and a definite but declining risk in the US. (Relative risk is an indicator of risk between two or more groups: a relative risk of 1 means there is no difference, a relative risk of 2 means there is double the risk.)

	Relative risk
US	1.3
Italy	2.0
Denmark	1.4
The Netherlands	1.5
UK	1.5
Sweden	1.2
Switzerland	1.3
China	2.3

Sources: 1. Tao S-C, Yu MC, Ross RK, Xiu K-W. Risk factors for breast cancer in Chinese women of Beijing. Int J Cancer 1988; 42: 495–8. 2. Van Loon AJM, Brug J, Goldbohm RA, van den Brandt P. Differences in cancer incidence and mortality among socioeconomic groups. Scand J Soc Med 1995; 23:110–20.

The information in Table 6.1 shows that the greater the difference in socioeconomic status between people in a given community the greater the difference in breast cancer risk. In other words, as access to education and income becomes more equal, the difference in breast cancer risk between the social classes also becomes more equal. For this reason the risk of breast cancer is reasonably equal among all social classes in the US, but is very different in the UK and China where there are substantial differences between the social classes.[23,24] In the US the difference in breast cancer mortality between social classes lessened steadily between 1969 and 1989.[25] This is partly due to an increase in breast cancer deaths in women of lower socioeconomic status and a fall in deaths in higher social class women.

The reasons for these trends can only be speculative, but it is likely that the differing risks for breast cancer among women of different social class is a reflection of differing nutritional experiences. It is possible that the increase in breast cancer among low social class groups is due to the fact that they now have access to a wider range of foods, including those previously consumed only by women of a higher income. The fall in breast cancer mortality among higher-income women which has been observed in some populations could largely be a result of the increased number of women with better education and higher income who are undergoing mammography examinations, thereby detecting breast cancer, and reducing the risk of early death, at an earlier stage.

However, changing patterns of other health-related behaviour among different social classes may also alter risk factors for breast cancer. These patterns include changes in fertility, alcohol consumption, exercise and food consumption. When all these factors are considered, however, it is the different food consumption patterns among social classes that is likely to be the most influential on the risk of breast cancer.

Struggling to find an explanation for these facts, I realised that there must be similar local Australian experiences that could offer some clues. There was no obvious starting point, except the official annual cancer statistics, which continued to show that breast cancer was more common among higher-income women. These statistics failed to supply an answer.

Scientific libraries are a magic resource if you can learn how to use them. We have such a library where I work, at the University of New South Wales, situated in an unpretentious area of south-east Sydney. It is a relatively new university and the book and journal collections cannot match those of the historic US and UK libraries. However, when the library was created during the 1940s, the librarians scoured the world for old publications and added them to the collection. It was to these 50 year old publications that I turned.

In these days of computer library searches the concept of browsing has been forgotten. Although it can be time-consuming, browsing can also be a surprisingly rewarding art form. I have generally found that it is only when I'm looking for nothing-in-particular that I find something-really-special in the endless corridors of long forgotten publications.

As every scientist knows, the thrill of discovery is something you have to experience, not just read about. Simple description betrays the real life excitement. I was enjoying a quiet Tuesday afternoon rifling through a section of outdated medical publications when one particular study, published way back in 1951, caught my eye. The author, Ross Patrick, happened to be an old aquaintance of mine. I met Ross Patrick, who was from Queensland, a state in northern Australia, years ago when he was a school medical officer. As part of his work Ross had gathered and recorded, in great detail, information about the heights and weights of the children within his jurisdiction, as well as details about their father's occupation.[26] In addition, he had compared this data with similar information collected as long ago as 1911.

This data showed that, on average, both boys and girls were about 4 inches (10 centimetres) taller and 20 pounds (about 9 kilos) heavier in 1951 than similar children in 1911. This experience has been observed in many populations. In addition, and of relevance to the search for the cause of breast cancer, the 12-year-old daughters of fathers with a professional occupation were on average 1 inch (2.5 centimetres) taller and 14 pounds (6.4 kilos) heavier than daughters of labourers. Similar surveys conducted in Queensland in 1976 (i.e. 25 years later than the 1951 surveys) showed that for Caucasian children these differences had disappeared.[27] However, for Aboriginal children, substantial differences in height and weight remained. Data is available from other surveys of Australian children and from international studies which strongly suggests that different nutritional experiences between social classes is the prime reason for the differences in height and weight.[28]

This discovery, made in a corner of the university library, although modest in the extreme in comparison with the great medical developments of the twentieth century, was a very exciting experience. The importance of Ross Patrick's information was the fact that when these children grew to adulthood, those taller and heavier girls of high socioeconomic status would experience higher risk of breast cancer than their shorter and thinner classmates.

An old friend, Ian Ring, who was head epidemiologist for the Queensland Health Department had also been interested in the social class and health status link. Following my request, he quickly gathered data which showed that 45–50-year-old Queensland women of high social class were at 10–20% increased risk of breast cancer. This was the age group that had been schoolchildren when Ross Patrick conducted his surveys. From a scientific perspective there are some reservations about the use of such data, but they are compatible with the findings shown in Table 6.1. The Queensland data are shown in Table 6.2. The information concerning correlations has been provided for specialist readers and shows that the data are reliable from a statistical perspective.

This information leads to a simple theory. **Breast cancer risk is associated with social class—the higher the social class the greater the risk**. Growth is intimately linked with nutritional experiences. Children of high social class have greater access to and consumption of a wider range of foods than children of lower social classes.

Table 6.2 Mean height and weight of 12-year-old Australian girls in 1950; age-standardised breast cancer mortality rates for Australian females 1984–88; by socioeconomic status

This data shows that schoolgirls from families of high socioeconomic status are taller and heavier than same-aged girls from families of low socioeconomic status. When the girls of high socioeconomic status become adults, they experience higher rates of breast cancer than other girls. It is speculated that these observations are a result of 'richer' nutritional experiences in the high-status girls.

Socioeconomic status	1	2	3	4	5
Height (cm)	153.3	150.9	150.5	151.6	150.3
Weight (kg)	47.2	41.1	41.2	40.6	40.6
Breast cancer mortality rate per 100 000	20	20	20	17	18

Source: May GMS, O'Hara VM, Dugdale AE. Patterns of growth in Queensland schoolchildren, 1911 to 1976. Medical Journal of Australia 1979; 2: 610–14.

Socioeconomic status according to father's occupation divided into quintiles. Highest to lowest—1 to 5. Correlation coefficients: socioeconomic status–height 0.69 (CI 0.49–0.98); socioeconomic status–weight 0.76 (CI 0.37–0.98); socioeconomic status–mortality rates 0.78 (CI 0.32–0.98).

Children of higher social classes are on average historically taller and heavier than children from lower social classes, in a particular community, because of these different nutritional experiences.[29] **Hence breast cancer risk may be associated with nutritional and growth experiences in childhood.**

These differences in childhood nutritional experiences may work in two ways:

1   by encouraging faster growth and hence more rapid division of cells, thus increasing the risk of a genetic mistake, or
2   by increasing weight and precipitating an early menarche.

This conclusion is supported by very recent US-based research (discussed earlier when we considered the association between height and risk of breast cancer) which shows that the earlier the age of achieving maximum height, the greater the risk of subsequent breast cancer, and that early-age maximum height also correlates with early age at menarche.[30]

While there is no knowledge available about the detailed mechanisms that are involved, these observations offer a rational explanation for the link between socioeconomic status and breast cancer that has puzzled doctors and other health workers for so many years.

These conclusions and observations also apply to Elizabeth. Her middle class family was genteel, highly educated, and brought up on fatty lamb, sausages, butter and jam. She drank abundant whole milk which, in Australia, was a government-provided, free of cost but compulsory mid-morning drink in all schools.

Elizabeth was in good company. Over the centuries, many other women with high-class backgrounds have developed breast cancer. Perhaps the most famous of all was the Empress Frederick of Prussia (Germany). She was the eldest daughter of Britain's Queen Victoria, wife of the Emperor of Prussia and mother of the infamous Kaiser Wilhelm II who led Germany into and out of World War I. Despite being short and having her first full-term pregnancy at the young age of 19 years, factors that should have reduced her breast cancer risk, she was diagnosed with advanced breast cancer soon after her 59th birthday. Her cancer was inoperable. She struggled on for nearly two years before she died in 1901. It is probable that she knew she had a lump in her breast but in those delicate times did not seek medical advice. The problem was not diagnosed until she was examined following a horse-riding mishap.

In our era it has become fashionable, and with good intention, for well known personalities of high social status to declare publicly that they have developed breast cancer. This includes the wives of former US presidents and the most famous film star of all, the wonderful Shirley Temple.

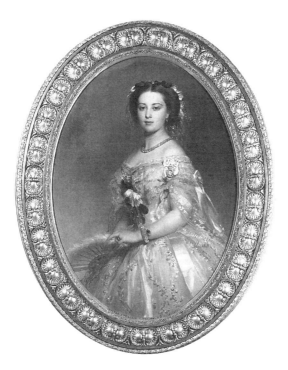

The 17-year-old Victoria, Princess Royal, was the eldest daughter of Queen Victoria and became the Empress Frederick of Prussia. Despite being short and becoming the mother of the future Kaiser Wilhelm II when she was only 19—both protective factors for breast cancer—she developed and died of breast cancer at 61 years of age.

Source: From the painting by Franz Winterhalter, 1857. The Royal Collection, copyright Her Majesty the Queen.

Exercise

Although the influence of exercise on the age at menarche is given special consideration in Chapter 7, a review of the general role of exercise in relation to breast cancer is presented here as there is some research which shows that regular exercise may reduce risk.

There appears to be no doubt that vigorous exercise during

childhood and adolescence depresses the production of ovarian hormones and hence defers the age at menarche, reducing to a small extent the subsequent risk of breast cancer.

However, there are mixed findings from studies of the influence of exercise in adults. Thune and colleagues working in Norway have produced convincing evidence that regular modest exercise offers equally modest protection from breast cancer.[31] This evidence has been supported by some recent large US-based studies[32] but not by other equally sound studies, also from the US.[33] Therefore we cannot come to any definite conclusions. However, in view of the sound evidence that large fluctuations in body weight during the postmenopausal years can increase breast cancer risk it is logical that exercise has some influence. This is because exercise uses energy, and weight fluctuations are in part a result of imbalances between energy input, that is, food consumption, and energy output, that is, exercise. Also, other important causes of ill health such as coronary heart disease are associated with a sedentary lifestyle.

A wise approach is to consider participating in regular physical exercise despite the absence of completely reliable evidence.

reproductive factors

The relationship between reproductive factors and breast cancer risk has been studied extensively and it is appropriate to consider these issues in some detail.

The influences of age at first birth, age at **menarche** (onset of menstruation) and age at menopause are well established.[1,2] As discussed above, early age at first birth reduces the risk of breast cancer by about half when women aged 20 years or less are compared with those aged 30 years or more; each year of early menarche increases breast cancer risk by 5–10%; and each year of deferral of menopause also increases risk by 5–10%.

At the turn of the century the average age at menarche in Western women was 14–16 years and menopause occurred at 42–46 years. The age at menarche has steadily declined and the age at menopause has risen throughout the twentieth century. These trends have been attributed to an increase in diet and a decline in physical activity.

For a woman born in Australia or the United States (or any Western country) in 1940, the average age at menarche would be 14 years. 'Early' menarche would mean that menstruation began 1–2 years before this age, and 'late' menarche 1–2 years after.

The same woman could expect menopause at 48–50 years. 'Early' menopause would occur at age 44–46 years and 'late' menopause at over 50 years.

---

menarche onset of menstruation

There are detailed records available from England and the United States dating back as far as 1830 which show that this decline in the age at menarche has been continuous for the past 150 years. This trend is similar for most Western countries and, in recent decades, also for Japan. Figure 7.1 illustrates the English and US data.

Figure 7.1 Age at menarche for US and UK girls over the past 160 years

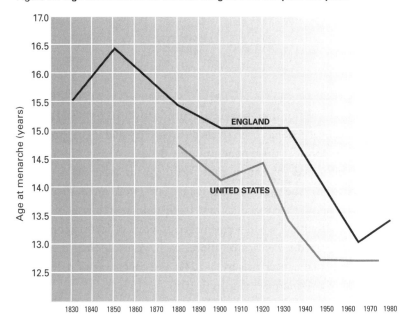

Source: Wyshak G, Frisch RE. Evidence for a secular trend in age of menarche. N Eng J Med 1982; 306:1033–5.

Age at menopause

It is accepted that late age at menopause increases the risk of breast cancer, although the reasons for the onset or deferral of menopause have not been determined. It is likely that both nutrition and exercise play a role. This view is based on the observation that early menopause is seen in populations with low food consumption and high exercise, such as China, and late menopause occurs in populations with high food and low exercise patterns, such as the United States. However, there is no direct evidence to support these conclusions.

The increased risk of breast cancer associated with early age of menarche and late age of menopause strongly suggests that the longer the exposure to sex hormones during the reproductive years, the higher the risk of breast cancer. This conclusion is supported by the experience of women who have had their ovaries surgically removed, most often because of cancer of the ovary. Such women experience substantially lower risk of breast cancer. Women who have both ovaries removed before the age of 40 years have a reduction in risk of about 50% compared with women who have a natural menopause.[3,4]

Studies in dogs, where data is readily available because of common breeding control practice, show that removal of the ovaries before the first oestrous cycle virtually eliminates the occurrence of breast cancer. It has also been shown that the fewer the oestrous cycles the dogs have had before removal of the ovaries, the lower the risk.[5] The important implication of these canine observations is the confirmation that breast cancer depends on the presence of sex hormones. This may be simplified: no sex hormones, no breast cancer.

While animal physiology may differ in some details from humans, the biology of all mammals, including humans, is very similar and many advances in knowledge have come from animal studies. Historically, cancer has been thought of as a disease confined to particular cells until Charles Huggins, an American surgeon and researcher, showed from his work on dogs and other mammals that many cancerous cells were only harmful if they existed in a sympathetic environment—such as female hormones in the case of breast cancer and male hormones in relation to prostate cancer. This led to the use of antihormone treatments, including removal of ovaries or testicles, and ultimately to antihormone pharmaceuticals such as tamoxifen, for the treatment and suppression of these cancers. Huggins was awarded the Nobel Prize for his pioneering work in this field. He died in 1996 at the age of 95 years.

These various findings—the increased risks of breast cancer associated with early age at menarche and late age at menopause, plus the experiences of women and dogs who have lost their ovaries—have led to the obvious conclusion that *the longer the exposure to sex hormones during the reproductive years the greater the risk.*

However, it is believed that the factors that are operating to increase the risk of breast cancer are likely to be much more complex than this. Early onset of menarche is also associated with much earlier establishment of regular ovulation and higher sex hormone levels than in girls with late onset of menarche.[6,7] We consider this in the next chapter on the age at menarche.

Age at first birth

One of the most consistent observations of breast cancer research is the reduced risk associated with increasing numbers of children. This phenomenon was studied as long ago as the 1920s. However, no one recognised that the important influence was not the number of children, but the age of the mother at her first full-term pregnancy. There appear to be two reasons for missing this crucial observation. First, in the US and Europe, where most of the research was conducted, few women had their first baby at a young age, even in the 1920s. Second, only the average ages of all women who gave birth were considered; such averages obscured substantial differences in breast cancer risk among women of different ages.

In 1970, a remarkable American epidemiologist from the Harvard School of Public Health, Brian MacMahon, showed clearly for the first time that women who have their first baby before the age of 18 years have only about one-third the breast cancer risk of those whose first birth is delayed until the age of 35 years or more.[8] He also showed that births after the first, even if they occur at a young age, have very little additional protective effect. The explanation for the reduced risk of breast cancer among women with many children is that they usually begin to have their many babies at a young age. MacMahon's careful studies involved observations of more than 12 000 women from seven countries—the US, the UK, Greece, Yugoslavia, Brazil, Taiwan and Japan. As this group of women included a wide range of ages, he was able to show not only the protective effect of early pregnancy but also the possible increase in risk that may be associated with late pregnancy.

These observations have been confirmed in many subsequent studies, perhaps the most important being *The Nurses Health Study* in the US.[9]

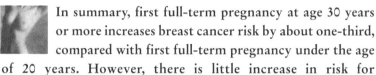 **In summary, first full-term pregnancy at age 30 years or more increases breast cancer risk by about one-third, compared with first full-term pregnancy under the age of 20 years. However, there is little increase in risk for pregnancies under the age of 28 years. The reason for the rapid increase in risk at about age 30 is not known.**

Over the years since MacMahon's original findings there has been continuous speculation about their meaning. MacMahon and his colleague Philip Cole originally suggested that complex oestrogen chemistry operating at an early adult age was behind the protective effect.[10] This theory may or may not be correct, but it stimulated research interest into the risk factors that operated in much earlier age groups than had been previously considered. A more likely explanation is the increased specialisation of breast cells late in pregnancy.[11] The breast cells are regarded as 'immature' before they specialise into milk-producing cells late in pregnancy. Such specialised cells are known to be less susceptible to **malignant** change than immature cells.

---

malignant having the potential for uncontrollable growth and spread

This latter theory has been tested in the laboratory with experimental rats by Jose Russo and colleagues working in Michigan.[11] Together with other workers they have been able to identify the actual cells in the rat breast that become malignant. They have also been able to show that cancer-initiating chemicals have a greater effect on rat breast cells that have not experienced the specialising effects of pregnancy. Experiences in experimental animals do not necessarily parallel similar experiences in humans, so Russo also grew human breast tissues in the laboratory from women with breast cancer. He confirmed that cancer-initiating chemicals had a lesser effect on more specialised human cells as well as in the experimental rats.

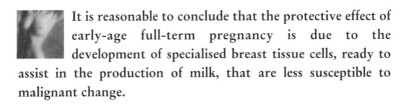

It is reasonable to conclude that the protective effect of early-age full-term pregnancy is due to the development of specialised breast tissue cells, ready to assist in the production of milk, that are less susceptible to malignant change.

However solid the evidence may be that early-age pregnancy offers substantial protection from breast cancer, it could be argued that this is of little practical value in today's society as few modern women have babies at an early age. Despite these reservations, if women were aware of this evidence, maybe some would choose not to defer pregnancy to an ever later age.

Elizabeth Sutherland had her first full-term baby at the age of 22 years, which should have offered her increased protection against breast cancer. In her case, perhaps other unknown factors overpowered this protective factor. One of these factors could have been genetics, as her mother's sister had died of breast cancer.

Number of births (parity)

It has long been recognised that women who have never had babies are at increased risk of breast cancer. The increase in risk is possibly as high as 50% in comparison with women who have had children. Seemingly in contradiction, there is also an increased risk of breast cancer for several years after a full-term pregnancy but, as discussed above, there is a reduced risk in the long term, particularly for women whose first pregnancy was at a young age. The contradiction is possibly due to the growth-enhancing properties of pregnancy hormones.[1]

Despite MacMahon's early findings, suggesting that the number of births after the first child did not affect the risk factor, there may be a small reduction in risk according to the number of full-term pregnancies beyond the first.[1] With the almost universal reduction in size of families in all societies it is unlikely that a definitive answer will ever be known. It is even more unlikely that modern women would choose to have more babies just to reduce slightly a theoretical chance of breast cancer.

Breastfeeding

Whether or not breastfeeding is associated with a change in risk of breast cancer has long been controversial. This is because various studies conducted in many countries have shown markedly different results. *The Nurses Health Study* (US) has not shown any association between breastfeeding and breast cancer.[12] On the other hand, studies from China show substantial reductions in risk associated with breastfeeding.[13,14]

The likely explanation for these conflicting findings is the duration of breastfeeding. Few US nurses breastfeed for longer than six months, compared with the many Chinese women who breastfeed for two or more years.

---

parity the number of births a woman has had

The reasons for any reduction in breast cancer risk associated with breastfeeding have to be speculative. A possible explanation is the reduction in ovulatory cycles and consequent reduction in oestrogen production associated with prolonged breastfeeding.

Given that Elizabeth breastfed her babies for an average of seven months for each child, the protection from breast cancer would have been very low compared with traditional Chinese mothers who received some protection from two to three years breastfeeding for each child. (The one-child policy has been effectively implemented in China since the 1970s. Most of the Chinese women with breast cancer who have been studied bore their children before this period.)

Breast milk

Interest in early life experiences and possible associations with breast cancer risk has led to a renewed interest in the influence that breast milk has on the risk of breast cancer in the infant—as distinct from breastfeeding and the risk of breast cancer in the mother.

In the 1950s and 1960s attempts were made to assess this issue. The stimulus for these studies was the search for a breast cancer 'virus', possibly transmitted by breast milk. No associations were found between breast cancer and consumption of breast milk. However, these were very simple studies.[15]

A recent study provides evidence on the intriguing question of whether a virus could be transmitted by breast milk to the daughters of mothers who later develop breast cancer. The answer appears to be—no. This was found in a very recent US-based study of 8299 women diagnosed with breast cancer.[15a]

Another study of women in New York has shown that women who were breastfed had about a 25% reduction in risk of breast cancer compared with women who were bottle-fed.[16] The reasons for this finding are speculative. Possibilities include the observation that bottle-fed babies born prior to the 1960s were considerably heavier and longer than breastfed babies (probably because of overfeeding with high-energy cow's milk). Cow's milk also contains a higher protein content as well as a high content of insulin-like growth factors that are found in cow's milk during the period after the birth of the calf. This may account for the faster growth and hence ultimate breast cancer risk in bottle-fed human babies.

Abortion

Many studies have attempted to find out whether either spontaneous or induced abortion is associated with breast cancer. An American research group, led by Professor Joel Brind of New York, has stated dogmatically that induced abortion (i.e. surgical or medically stimulated abortion) as distinct from naturally occurring abortion is a significant independent risk factor for breast cancer.[17] This opinion is based on a careful meta-analysis, or review, of all 23 research studies that have examined this issue. Yet this opinion, which is based on accepted research criteria and methodology, is almost certainly wrong. This major error is probably due to the difficulty the research studies would have had in determining the exact number of abortions that occur in a given population, particularly where there are legal sanctions against abortion. Legal sanctions, plus the great sensitivity associated with abortion in many countries, appears to have led to a consistent undercounting of the number of induced abortions among the healthy (i.e. no breast cancer) control group. This undercounting, plus use of the less reliable case-control study method (almost all 23 studies were case-control studies), biased the results of this extensive review of previous research studies and led to the unwarranted inference that such abortions increase subsequent risk of breast cancer.

For this reason a recently completed study in Denmark is of particular value.[18] There is a universal identification system in Denmark that involves mandatory reporting of abortions, thus allowing an accurate count of the number of cases of abortion. This enormous Danish study involved over 1.5 million women and

370 000 abortions, and included more than 10 000 women with breast cancer. The study has not shown any link between induced abortions and the risk of breast cancer.

 Accordingly, women should not worry about the risk of breast cancer when termination of pregnancy is being considered.

The nuns' story

THE LIFE OF A NUN attracts both peculiar fascination and supportive admiration from the greater community. Living a life of celibacy, their dedication to God requires that they never marry and never have children. It hardly seems fair, given their sacrifices and devotion, that nuns should be one of the highest-risk groups in terms of breast cancer.

For over 200 years, members of Christian, particularly Catholic, religious orders have been subjected to research studies aimed at determining whether the religious life had a role in causing or preventing diseases. It is perhaps of passing interest that virtually all those conducting the research have been men, many of them members of religious orders themselves.

The earliest known study of nuns was conducted as long ago as 1713 by the Italian, Ramazzini, who was the first to make the observation that breast cancer was common in nuns. He accurately, and remarkably, related the cause to celibacy. In 1842, another Italian, Rigoni-Stern, compared the patterns of cancer in nuns from Verona with married women. He found that breast cancer was nearly ten times more common in nuns than in married women, but that cancer of the uterus was twice as common in married women than in nuns. The reason for this latter observation was not to unfold until the 1980s.

During the next century the interest in nuns continued unabated, particularly when it was discovered that their deaths due to tuberculosis were appallingly high and well in excess of the general community. Again, the reason—living in close proximity and thereby spreading the bacillus by coughing, plus the added effect of poor diets— would take many years to become apparent.

It was not until 1949 that Versluys, working in Holland, showed that the pattern of cancer seen in nuns was not due to their religious lifestyle but to their status as single celibate women. He did this simply by comparing the data for nuns with the data for other single women.

After a gap of 100 years, in 1950, the observation that cancer of the uterine cervix was rare in nuns was made again, this time in relation to French-Canadian nuns.

During the 1950s a religious father, Francis Madigan, collected data about nuns from 41 religious communities in the United States (Figure 7.2). He found that deaths due to breast cancer were nearly twice as common, compared with married women of the same age. As the two groups got older, the differences increased—by the age of 80 years, deaths due to breast cancer were three times greater among nuns than among married women. These patterns of death from breast cancer in nuns and married women are almost identical to those observed in Italy two centuries earlier.

It took all that time for the reasons for the different rates of death due to breast and cervical cancer to become apparent.[19]

Figure 7.2 Breast cancer death rate (per 1000) of nuns, compared with same-age married women. The graph shows the much greater death rate from breast cancer among nuns compared with married women. The main reason is the protection against breast cancer provided by early-age first full-term pregnancy among the married women. This protection was not available to members of celibate religious orders.

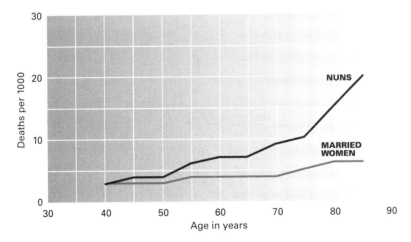

Source: Fraumeni JF, Lloyd JW., Smith EM, Wagoner JK. Cancer mortality among nuns: role of marital status in etiology of neoplastic disease in women. J Natl Cancer Inst 1969; 42: 455–68.

With respect to breast cancer, we now know the key factor is the protection offered by early full-term pregnancy. In the case of cervical cancer, the key factor is the sexually transmitted human papilloma virus, the same family of viruses that causes common warts.

Age at menarche

We have discussed earlier the influence of age at **menarche** on breast cancer risk but, in view of constantly emerging new research findings, the link demands our renewed attention.

Menarche, or onset of menstruation, is a very delicate time for young females. It is a clear step from girlhood to womanhood.

It was first thought that delayed menarche was primarily due to exercise. This was largely because of the common observation that girls who engaged in strenuous activity, such as ballet dancing, swimming or running, showed considerable delay in the onset of the menses. It was to be several decades before the main determinant of age at menarche—nutrition—was recognised.

There are marked differences in the age at menarche in different populations. Traditional Chinese, Japanese and southern African girls experience menarche at 17 years of age or even later, in contrast to Western girls who may be as young as 11 years. Not only is the age at menarche different, the underlying sex hormone chemistry is different. The temptation has been to conclude that ethnicity or **genetics** is the obvious reason for these differences—but the fact that Japanese-American girls, whose families have lived in the United States for several generations, are of similar height and weight and have similar age at menarche to Caucasian-American girls clearly demonstrates that it is environmental, most probably nutritional, factors that influence these events.[20]

A combined American and South African research team, led by

menarche start of menstruation
genetics heredity

Hill and Wynder of New York, demonstrated the dramatic differences between adolescent girls from a traditional society—the Bantu people of South Africa—and similar aged girls from a fully developed industrial society—New York.[21] The New York (Caucasian) girls were, on average, 11 centimetres taller and 12 kilograms heavier and experienced menarche more than two years earlier than the Bantu girls. The diets of the New York girls had 25% more calories, double the fat and animal protein and 30% less carbohydrates and vegetable proteins than the Bantu girls. In addition, sex hormone serum (blood) levels were significantly higher in the New York girls. A different group of well nourished Bantu girls living in a reserve has been observed to have early-age menarche, further adding to the conclusion that the initiation of menarche is affected by nutrition.[22] As adults, New York girls are at high risk, and Bantu girls at low risk, of breast cancer. There is an average increase in risk of breast cancer of about 5% for each year of decrease in age at menarche.[23] The marked difference in sex hormone levels between the Bantu and New York girls has also been shown between rural Chinese and British women.[24] The age at menarche in the Chinese is as late as 17 years and for the British 12 to 13 years. The British women have up to 50% higher oestrogen and testosterone (female and male hormones) serum concentrations than their Chinese counterparts. British women are much taller and heavier, and have six times the breast cancer risk of their Chinese counterparts.

This very late age at menarche in Chinese and Bantu females is similar to that for Britain in 1865—that is, nearly 150 years ago! Since that time there has been a decrease in age at menarche by an average of 3–4 months each decade in the UK and in other developed nations such as the US, Australia and Sweden. It is of interest that the downward trend in the UK has quite recently been replaced by a trend in the opposite direction.[25] The reason for this reversal of decreasing age at menarche is not known but may be due to fashion-oriented dieting; anorexia nervosa has increased and is a known cause of menstrual disturbance.[26]

Rose Frisch is a research scientist who has spent her professional life exploring the biology of menarche at the Harvard Center for Population Studies in Cambridge, Massachusetts. Among her wide range of discoveries, two stand out in the breast cancer story. The first was in 1972 when she showed that both well nourished and undernourished girls of British extraction, living in Alabama, experienced menarche when they reached the same weight, despite the fact that the well nourished girls were on average two years younger than the undernourished girls.[27] The menarche has been related to a constant weight, 46 kilograms, and height, about 155 centimetres, for over a century. From an evolutionary perspective, the regulation of female size at sexual maturity has obvious survival advantages for the human species: birth weight and pre-pregnancy maternal weight are correlated, and infant survival is correlated with birth weight.

Rose Frisch's second major contribution is her work on exercise and menstruation. She formally confirmed the popular observation that athletes, ballet dancers and other girls who exercise vigorously experience deferment of the menarche.[29] She also showed there was a lower risk of breast cancer in women who had trained as athletes at a young age.[29] The mechanism by which exercise influences menstruation and thereby ovulation is not known. It is speculated that a minimal balance between energy input and output is required for the onset and continuation of ovulation—in other words, a balance between food consumption and exercise.

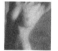 **Since Rose Frisch's early research there have been many studies which have shown that moderate exercise during adult life is associated with a probable reduction in breast cancer risk.[30,31] However, the evidence is conflicting and we shall have to return to this issue.**

The extent of the exercise and the level and composition of food consumption required to alter the age at menarche or to reduce the risk of breast cancer are not known in detail. However, there is sound evidence that consumption of meat, compared with vegetables, nuts and cereals, will reduce the age at menarche by about 12 months and thereby modestly increase the subsequent risk of breast cancer.[32] Therefore, a diet of low-fat foods (cereals, fruit and vegetables, and meat used as a garnish rather than the main item) is to be encouraged during childhood. This advice is consistent with most national dietary guidelines.

Although to most people the evidence gathered by Rose Frisch and others is sufficient to establish the conclusions outlined above, in the scientific world this is still indirect evidence and therefore not good enough. Hence the need for prospective direct evidence. Prospective evidence has greater validity than retrospective evidence because observations are made before outcomes are known and hence there is much less opportunity for bias. While few would suspect scientists of being biased, unconsciously, like everyone else, they wish to see successful results and therefore tend to find what they are looking for. Similarly, patients who are participating in a research study can easily bias the results because they tend to seek to please the questioners.

For these reasons two groups of researchers, one from Quebec City and the other from Harvard (including that great contributor to the breast cancer story, Brian MacMahon), initiated prospective studies aimed at identifying the role of diet in young girls in breast cancer events that may not become clinical cancer for 40–60 years. More than two hundred 9 and 10 year old girls were recruited into each of the studies and their diet, growth and menstrual experiences were observed for six years.[33,34] The results of the two studies were broadly similar and confirmed the many other non-prospective studies. The results showed there was a direct connection between body weight and age at menarche, and taller and fatter girls menstruated well before thin and short girls. Age at menarche was not associated with particular levels of consumption of energy, protein, fat or carbohydrate.

We finish consideration of the age at menarche with some theoretical issues concerning patterns of ovulation.

First, it has been found that females with later age at menarche are more likely to have **anovular** (no ovulation) cycles than females with early menarche and, in turn, the populations at highest risk for breast cancer have the highest frequency of ovulatory cycles.[35]

Second, in 1983 two Finnish scientists, Dan Apter and Reijo Vihko,[36] confirmed that girls with early onset of menarche establish ovulatory cycles at an earlier age than girls with late onset of menarche. They also demonstrated that, even in early puberty, before menarche, those girls who were to experience early menarche had higher serum sex hormones than girls whose menarche took place after the age of 13 years. Girls with early menarche were also characterised by high circulating sex hormone concentrations for some years after menarche.

Third, in a recent large US-based study[37] led by Michels-Blanck, it has been shown that irregular menstruation at age 20 years is associated with a modest reduction in breast cancer risk. This study confirms previous similar findings.[38,39]

The mechanisms behind these various influences on menstrual patterns are not known but again early dietary experiences are under suspicion.

Unfortunately, with the exception of the need to reduce meat consumption, this wide range of studies does not give precise answers to the questions we need to ask: how much food, what types of food and how much exercise are appropriate for children during the **perimenarcheal** period? This is the problem with breast cancer—there are so many tantalising clues but few definite answers. However, we must struggle on.

Elizabeth had her first period at 12 years of age. This would have substantially (by about 25%) increased her risk of breast cancer compared with Chinese or Japanese girls. Her early age at menarche

---

anovular when no ovulation occurs
perimenarcheal around the time of menarche

was probably due to two factors: her 'rich' diet as a child, and her dislike of physical sports activities. She was of course in this respect very similar to most other Western girls of the period.

The Pill and hormone replacement therapy

There is obvious concern that the use of hormones such as the contraceptive Pill to prevent pregnancy, or hormone replacement therapy to prevent the onset of osteoporosis and maintain female physiology after the menopause, could lead to increased risk of breast cancer. A great many studies have been performed to explore these issues.

Even a small increase in risk of breast cancer associated with such hormone use is important because of the frequency of the exposure, which involves many millions of women on a worldwide basis. The technique of **meta-analysis**, combining the results from more than 50 studies on breast cancer and use of the Pill, has fortunately shown only a small increase in risk (by about 20%) even for long-term users.[40] This increase in risk gradually reduces to nil, 10 years after ceasing use of the oestrogen/progestin combination.

Despite these findings, which were based almost wholly on studies that compared two groups of women—one group with breast cancer and one free of breast cancer—there have been suspicions that there may have been some increase in risk in young women who used oral contraceptives prior to first pregnancy or for prolonged periods.

Yet, again, *The Nurses Health Study*, from Harvard University, has provided confirmatory evidence using the more reliable prospective study method, where large numbers of women were observed over 15 years. They were able to demonstrate that there was no increase in

---

meta-analysis review of a number of studies

risk of breast cancer even among women over 40 years of age who had used oral contraceptives for 10 or more years.[41] They did not have sufficient data to examine the risk for women under the age of 40 years. These findings are in accord with the few other reliable prospective studies, the most recent of which is a large study of more than 62 000 Dutch women.[42] The Dutch study also showed that oral contraceptive use was safe, except for women with a first-degree relative (mother or sister) with breast cancer. The risk was raised by about 50% among these women.

These findings should give reasonable, but not complete, security to women who use oral contraceptives. However, we need additional studies of younger women and women with a family history of breast cancer before oral contraceptives can be given absolute guarantees of safety.

The story of postmenopausal hormone therapy is not the same as for oral contraceptive hormone use, as there appears to be an increase in risk of breast cancer of about 40% after 10 years use of such hormones. This conclusion is based on *The Nurses Health Study*, which measures and observes events in very well fed, well educated American women.[43] Such women are typical of middle class women of the Western World but certainly not of Asian and eastern countries. With respect to health, the main differences between women of these two worlds is diet.

There are many difficulties when seeking to measure the effects of hormone replacement therapy. Not only are populations of users different—the content, method of delivery and length of use may all be different. Hormone replacement therapy (HRT) is used as oestrogen alone, oestrogen combined with progestin, and progestin alone. The HRT may be delivered by a pill or a skin patch, or even an implant of the hormone under the skin. The method of delivery of HRT alters the rate and level of absorption of the hormones into the body and probably has some effect on the influence of the HRT. For example, there is incomplete evidence that HRT delivered by skin patch does not cause the weight gain that can be associated with oral

HRT. *The Nurses Health Study* has also shown that the elevated risk of breast cancer is no different whether HRT is given as oestrogen alone or in combination with progestin. (This is in contrast to cancer of the body of the uterus where the addition of progestins does oppose the effect of oestrogen which when given alone increases risk.)

These findings with respect to HRT and breast cancer have not been confirmed by the similar large prospective study in Holland, where no increase in risk has been identified.[42] The follow-up of participants in the Dutch study is only 3–4 years compared with the 20 year follow up in *The Nurses Health Study*, and so we cannot have the same level of confidence in the findings.

To complicate the story further, the latest findings (June 1997) from *The Nurses Health Study* bring good news.[42] Deaths from all causes, including the increase in mortality from breast cancer, are reduced by more than one-third (about 37%) among nurses using HRT. This is due mainly to a reduction in cardiovascular disease. **Cardiovascular disease** is the formal name for sclerosis (thickening) of the coronary arteries, the arteries to the brain and to the arteries that circulate blood around the body. HRT certainly reduces by about 40% the incidence of coronary heart disease (i.e. 'heart attacks') and possibly reduces strokes by about the same proportion. The data is not reliable with respect to strokes because the studies on HRT have all been in relatively younger women who are at low risk of stroke.

Finally, and regretfully, a new problem with HRT has just emerged.[44] It has been discovered that use of HRT at the time of mammographic screening increases the density of breast tissue. This increase in breast tissue density obscures the shadow in the X-ray pictures caused by early breast cancer tumours and lowers the chance of detecting the cancer. This has been shown to increase the rate of discovery of breast cancer *between* mammography screenings. The phenomenon has become so well recognised that it even has a name—'interval cancer'. Given the benefits of both mammography and HRT for many women, there is no obvious solution except to advise all women who participate in

---

cardiovascular disease thickening of the arteries

mammography programs to continue breast self- and clinical examinations despite clearance by mammography. In other words, mammography is absolutely *not* infallible.

Postmenopausal hormone therapy, or hormone replacement therapy (HRT), carries many benefits, the most important being the reduced risk of **osteoporosis** and cardiovascular disease (heart attack and stroke). There does not appear to be an additional increase in risk of breast cancer (above the 40% referred to) for women with a family history of breast cancer and use of HRT.[43]

Given the findings that there does appear to be some increased risk of breast cancer associated with long-term HRT, women in the postmenopausal age group will feel a well justified concern. The most appropriate advice is that each woman's situation should be individually assessed. When my wife, Margaret, read of the increase in risk of breast cancer of about 40% associated with use of HRT for five or more years, she immediately stopped the therapy because, she said, 'I would rather drop dead from a heart attack than get breast cancer.' So the choice is very personal.

We then asked 100 female health professionals aged 30–50 years of age: 'Would you rather have breast cancer or a heart attack?' The response was extraordinary—90% of the women chose to have a heart attack in preference to breast cancer. These health professionals are not, of course, representative of the community—they are very well informed and experienced in medical issues—but it is clear that women have a fear of breast cancer that is quite different from their fears about other medical matters.

There are reasons other than health issues for women to consider using hormone replacement therapy. The menopause is a vulnerable time for many women. They may feel that their body 'will fall apart', as was expressed by a 55 year old physician who was participating in our postgraduate public health program. Loss of skin and muscle tone may be a worry. Postmenopausal women may also be concerned about their relationship with spouse or partner, for good reason— the media are full of stories of older men successfully gaining new, much

---

osteoporosis fragile bones due to calcium loss

younger partners. This can all lead to a major loss of self-confidence. HRT can help overcome these problems.

In these circumstances, no specific guide can be offered with respect to HRT. For many women it may be worth considering the use of HRT for about five years after the menopause. Such use will give some relief from the symptoms of the menopause, and female characteristics that are hormone-dependent will be retained for an additional period. The risks from breast cancer are quite small for such limited use.

The best advice is to seek an individual assessment from your doctor. If you are aware of the information outlined above, you will be in a good position to have an informed discussion and to come to a rational decision.

These observations again warn of the need to consider issues from a global perspective. Virtually all the studies of HRT and postmenopausal breast cancer have been conducted in Western countries where women are at high risk of cardiovascular diseases. Therefore, as suggested above, the increased risk of breast cancer associated with HRT is perhaps acceptable because of the increased protection HRT provides against cardiovascular disease. But this 'balance of risk' does not apply in Asian countries such as Japan, Korea and China, where cardiovascular disease is not a major issue, although it is increasing.

As always, there is another qualification: osteoporosis (fragile bones, associated with decalcification during older age) is probably more common in Asian than in Western women, possibly because of lower calcium intake in their diet, and there is no doubt that HRT is by far the most effective preventive influence on osteoporosis. This is another reason for assessing the needs of women for HRT on an individual basis.

8

from atom bombs to alcohol

Atom bombs

The year of 1945 is of great historical significance. World War II ended for Europeans during May of that year but continued for those fighting in the Pacific war. It was feared that the struggle between the Americans and the Japanese would go on for years—until two atom bombs were exploded, destroying the cities and the inhabitants of Hiroshima and Nagasaki. A war that had lasted for nearly six years was over.

In 1951 the Atomic Bomb Casualty Commission, a cooperative Japan–US research organisation (now known as the Radiation Effects Research Foundation), was set up. With its headquarters in Hiroshima this remarkable joint venture has carefully traced as many of the survivors' lives as possible, observing in detail their health and social well-being.[1]

For people investigating breast cancer a vital clue has been revealed. Age of exposure to atomic radiation has been found to be a key to breast cancer risk. Young women who were exposed to the same amount of radiation as older women were found to suffer a far greater risk of breast cancer. For those who were exposed before the age of five years, there was nearly a tenfold increase in the risk of subsequent breast cancer when compared with those who were over the age of 40 years at the time of exposure. These observations are shown in Figure 8.1.

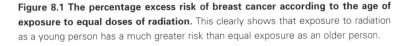

Figure 8.1 The percentage excess risk of breast cancer according to the age of exposure to equal doses of radiation. This clearly shows that exposure to radiation as a young person has a much greater risk than equal exposure as an older person.

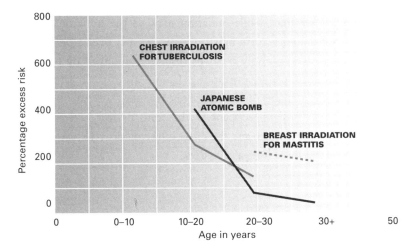

Sources: | McGregor DH, Land CE, Choi K, et al. Breast cancer incidence among atomic bomb survivors, Hiroshima and Nagasaki, 1950–69. J Natl Cancer Inst 1977; 59: 799–811. 2. Miller AB, Howe GR, Sherman GJ, et al. Mortality from breast cancer after irradiation during fluoroscopic examinations in patients being treated for tuberculosis. N Engl J Med 1989; 321: 1285–9. 3. Land CE, Boice JD, Shore RE, et al. Breast cancer risk from low-dose exposures to ionising radiation: results of parallel analysis of three exposed populations of women. J Natl Cancer Inst 1980; 65: 353–68.

Another important new concept also followed the atomic disaster. Studies showed that this increased risk of breast cancer could continue for up to 50 years (so far) after the initial exposure to radiation and that, although such exposure to radiation increased the risk of breast cancer, it did not bring forward the age of breast cancer development. Young girls who experienced atomic radiation in Hiroshima developed breast cancer in their fifth or later decade, exactly the same age as other Japanese women who were not exposed. However, the proportion of the girls from Hiroshima who developed breast cancer was ten times greater than that of unexposed counterparts.

These experiences suggest that any increased risk of breast cancer associated with radiation may persist throughout life.

One subsidiary concept is that, although the initiation of the increased risk of breast cancer was clearly due to the atomic radiation, females retained their virtual monopoly of the disease compared with males. It follows that, while radiation may be the initiator of the increased risk, other factors must influence events over a period of many years. The monopoly over the disease maintained by females suggests that the prime promoting factor, as distinct from the initiating factor, remains the female sex hormones.

A second subsidiary concept is the long period between the initiating factor, radiation, and the onset of the disease. This so-called *latent period* can be as long as 50 years.

Radiation

The atomic bomb story was to repeat itself in the form of medical treatments. Despite the knowledge that radiation from any source increased the risk of many types of cancers, radiation was freely used after the war years for a range of non-life-threatening medical conditions. Radiation-based treatments included therapy for inflammation of the breast after the birth of a baby, alleged enlargement of the thymus gland in childhood (a condition that is no longer recognised as ever existing), tinea of the scalp in babies, scoliosis (a spinal condition in teenagers) and X-rays for tuberculosis. The experience has been the same as for the atom bomb—the younger the age of exposure to radiation the greater the subsequent risk of breast cancer.[2-4] Many older readers will recall the fitting of shoes under the active guidance of X-ray machines at the front of the local shoe shop. I am unaware of any formal studies showing that such practices increased breast cancer risk, although it is an obvious possibility.

Despite the very low doses of radiation involved in these treatments, the rates of breast cancer as adult women increased three to four times above that of women who had not had such radiation treatment as young girls.

Disregarding the power we gain from hindsight, it seems outrageous that radiation was so widely used as a treatment on men, women and children. There was no verification of its value, the conditions being treated were of unknown cause and the method had been established as dangerous since the days, and the adverse personal experiences, of Marie Curie and others at the turn of the century.

Today, radiation remains a widely used form of treatment. Although the risks remain the same, the benefits are far more understood. As a medical intervention its use is considered according to the balance between risk and benefit. Mammography, aimed at the early detection of breast cancer, is a classic example. There is no doubt about the value of radiation for the detection of breast cancer, but the radiation exposure of mammography imposes a small cumulative risk of increased breast cancer, particularly for those women who have annual examinations. At the present, our level of knowledge indicates that the benefits of mammography far outweigh the risks, and therefore it is acceptable to advise mammographical examination.

Alcohol

Alcohol, particularly the overconsumption of alcohol, takes the blame for a number of our medical as well as our social problems. Yet how could alcohol have anything to do with a woman's breasts?

The bad news is that not only is there a suspicion that alcohol consumption may raise the risk of breast cancer, but the evidence is well established.[5-9]

 Alcohol is almost certainly a strong factor in the increase in the risk of breast cancer.

It is believed that regular consumption of alcohol increases the risk by about 10–20%. It is still uncertain what quantities of alcohol are responsible and whether the age of drinking has an impact.

The possibility that there could be a link between alcohol and breast cancer arose from a chance observation by RR Williams and his colleague, JW Horm, who were conducting surveys of the US population in the 1970s for the National Cancer Institute.[8] Their findings did not create interest and years were to pass before the scientific community recognised the significance of this observation. Again, with the advantage of hindsight it is easy to be critical. But it is in the tradition of research to be careful and not to make unjustified claims. This philosophy is based on long experience and the bitter lessons of thalidomide and other medications that have gone horribly wrong.

Then suddenly, in the 1980s, research into this issue began in earnest. More than 50 formal research studies were conducted throughout the world during the 1980s and 1990s in an effort to determine what role, if any, alcohol played in relation to breast cancer. The primary reason for such effort was the dawning realisation that, if alcohol was shown to be a risk factor for breast cancer, it would be the only readily modifiable risk factor so far identified.

Matthew Longnecker, a young American epidemiologist from California, had developed an interest in the issue during the 1980s. His early work tended to confirm the link between alcohol consumption and some increase in the risk of breast cancer.[5] But the many other studies on this issue tended to confuse rather than clarify the picture. In 1994, Longnecker applied the newly developing technique of meta-analysis to the many studies that had so quickly become available.[6] Meta-analysis had been developed many years earlier by researchers in the education field but the approach had not been recognised by their counterparts in health.

In essence, the technique is simple. The results from all the studies are added together and an average of the outcomes is calculated. But there are problems, the most important being that there is no way of excluding poorly conducted studies without creating serious bias. In addition, studies carried out in rich countries may not be valid in poor countries due to the difference in diet, exercise, fertility and other environmental factors—all of which may influence the risk of breast cancer in any particular population. Despite these reservations, if the procedures are used in a common-sense manner the results can be very helpful, and Longnecker's meta-analysis is considered confirmation of the link between alcohol and breast cancer. The analysis also showed that the more you drank the greater the risk. Put simply, Longnecker was able to show that one drink each day increased the risk of breast cancer by about 10%, while three drinks each day upped the risk to nearly 30%. However, the issue of age at which regular drinking of alcohol commenced was not resolved.

Despite the inevitable criticisms that go with the role of a great international power, the United States has made an unique, and largely unknown, contribution to humanity through the work of its vast research organisations. While the issue of age-related alcohol and breast cancer risk is far from major in the context of other health issues, in 1990 workers at the US National Cancer Institute again began to explore the alcohol and breast cancer problem. Christine Swanson, another epidemiologist from the Cancer Institute, led a large team that began to examine the lifetime personal drinking habits of hundreds of women with diagnosed breast cancer from New Jersey, Georgia and Washington State.

By 1997 they were able to confirm (in principle) Longnecker's key findings.[7] **They found that nearly 14 drinks per week, that is, two per day, were needed to substantially increase the risk.** In addition, they found no relation between breast cancer and early-age drinking patterns, and came to the conclusion that the main effects of alcohol were as a promoter in the late stages of the years it takes for the full development of breast cancer. These emerging insights into the influence of alcohol on the risk of breast cancer have been recently reviewed by bringing together the results of six prospective studies from the US, Canada, the Netherlands and Sweden.[9] When combined, these prospective studies involved 322 647 women over an 11 year period and therefore the outcome can be regarded as very reliable. This review again confirmed that for each alcohol drink each day there was an increased risk of breast cancer of 9–10%.

It seems highly unlikely that alcohol is an initiator of breast cancer. The possible mechanism for its effect is oestrogen metabolism in the body. This has been shown in a special study of women who consumed two drinks of alcohol each day.[10] This amount of alcohol was associated with an increase in oestrogen levels in the blood and oestrogen, as you now know, is essential for the development of breast cancer.

As with most risk factors for diseases of all types, it is unwise to consider a single disease in isolation. While it is highly likely that two or more alcoholic drinks per day increase the risk of breast cancer, such modest (some readers may regard such consumption levels as being immodest!) consumption also reduces the risk of coronary heart disease, which remains the single most important disease for older Western women (over 55 years).[11,12] This reduction of coronary heart disease is of about the same magnitude as the increase in risk of breast cancer associated with moderate consumption of alcohol.

There is sufficient research evidence to conclude that alcohol consumption increases the risk of breast cancer. This conclusion allows the development of formal prevention policies and approaches which take into account both the benefits and the harm associated with alcohol consumption. On the benefit side there is the known reduction in coronary heart disease plus, of course, the great pleasure that many of us gain from drinking wine, beer and other alcoholic beverages. On the harm side are the well known problems of liver and brain damage plus increased risk of traffic accidents and domestic violence.

 A reasonable guideline is to limit alcohol consumption to a maximum of two drinks per day.

Elizabeth, as the daughter of a Methodist clergyman, could have been expected to rebel and to have started drinking too much alcohol at parties and local social gatherings. She disliked the taste of beer but, as a married woman, she drank the two glasses of wine each evening that had become fashionable in Australia.

world war II and leftist tendencies

Wartime food shortages and breast cancer

When looking for possibilities for the prevention of breast cancer, I came across a single paragraph in an obscure article by Steinar Tretli which described the retardation in growth of Norwegian schoolchildren during the 1940s wartime occupation of Norway.[1] I later learned that another Norwegian, LJ Vatten, had made a similar suggestion.[2] Both suggested that Norway might provide the opportunity to test the hypothesis that reduction in food consumption during childhood may lead to reduced rates of breast cancer.

I checked through the computer-based list of publications to see if either Tretli or Vatten had followed up this idea, but nothing came up on the screen. So I wrote to Tretli's group in Oslo who sent a reply saying that they were about to publish a paper that showed a reduction in the incidence of breast cancer as had been predicted.[3] However, they did not appear to have followed the patterns of *deaths* from breast cancer (as distinct from **incidence**). Deaths are probably a more accurate indicator of trends with respect to breast cancer because of the impact of mammography. Mammographies artificially increase the incidence of breast cancer by making the diagnosis several years earlier than would otherwise be the case. Even death

incidence the extent of occurrence of a disease in a given population

rates are a problem when making comparisons over the years because improved treatment methods also alter the pattern.

So I reviewed the death patterns for young Norwegian women in the World Health Organisation Annual Statistics Reports and, sure enough, for those Norwegian women who were 10 or so years of age during the early war years there was a fall in the expected number of deaths due to breast cancer 30 years later. This is important information because it provides a natural experiment that could not be conducted by artificial means.

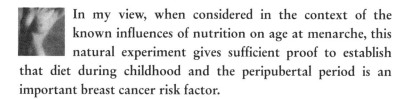 **In my view, when considered in the context of the known influences of nutrition on age at menarche, this natural experiment gives sufficient proof to establish that diet during childhood and the peripubertal period is an important breast cancer risk factor.**

The breast cancer story in Norway is an extraordinary one. Before the German forces swept into Norway in 1940, many food supplies, particularly meats and dairy products, were imported. These imports were to be virtually eliminated for the four hard years of the war. Dieticians have not generally been recognised for their bravery under fire but in Norway a courageous group, under the very noses of the Nazis, began secretly to record the detailed dietary experiences of 20–30 Oslo families. The types and amounts of food consumed for each meal were noted plus the details of their daily work and activities for the whole of the war years. In addition, the school health service kept up their supervision of children, whether or not medical and other supplies were available. These records survived the war.[4,5]

The Oslo families experienced a 25% daily reduction in average caloric (energy) intake during this four year period. This fall in calories was due mainly to substantially reduced consumption (by about 50%) of animal-based fats. The consumption of animal protein fell by about 20% and total protein by 15%. The adverse impact of this reduction in nutrition is confirmed by a reduction in the average height of all age groups of children and adolescents from Oslo during the war years.[6] This is shown with respect to 12-year-old Norwegian girls in Figure 9.1.

Figure 9.1 Heights of 12-year-old Norwegian schoolgirls. There was an approximate reduction in average height of about 5% among females who were aged 8-17 years during the war years. This reduction in height was almost certainly due to restrictions on available food during their growth years.

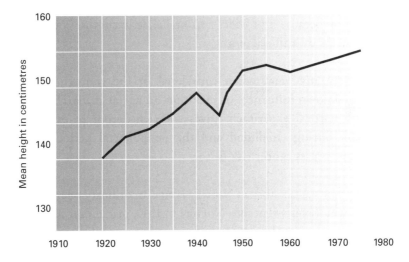

Source: Bruntland GH, Liestol K, Walloe L. Height, weight and menarcheal age of Oslo schoolchildren during the last 60 years. Ann Human Biol 1980; 7: 307–22.

In 1945 there was a fall in average height of 1–2 centimetres for all ages from 8–17 years, compared with average height in 1940. In 1947 average heights for these age groups increased or equalled those for 1940. Norwegian females who were children or teenagers during 1941–45, and who had such a reduced caloric intake, experienced a 19.3% reduction in breast cancer mortality rates in 1980–85 as 45–54 year old women, as compared with those females who were teenagers before or after the war years. The breast cancer mortality rates for 45–54 year old women in 1986–92 were higher than the pre-1980 rates. This age group of women would mostly have been children or teenagers after the war years. These data are shown in Figure 9.2. The

Figure 9.2 Breast cancer mortality rates per 100 000 Norwegian women aged 45–54 years for 5 year periods, 1950–92. This graph shows there was an approximate reduction of 19% in expected death rates due to breast cancer among those who were children or teenagers during the war years when food supplies were restricted. The implication is that restriction of food during childhood and adolescence retards growth and defers the age of onset of menarche, both of which may reduce subsequent breast cancer risk.

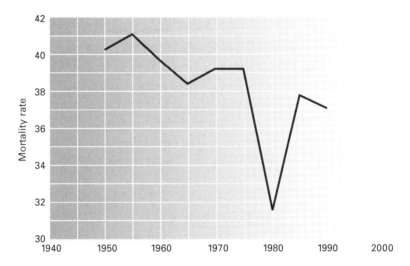

Sources: World Health Statistics Annuals 1950–94, WHO Geneva.

correlation between height and later breast cancer mortality rate is reliable (statistically significant).

With the exception of Holland,[8] these experiences are different from other European countries that also had high prewar breast cancer rates but no reduction in breast cancer among females who were teenagers during the war. The explanation is probably that, contrary to popular belief, the nutritional status of the whole community, as compared with sections of the community, actually improved during the war years. For example, in the United Kingdom the average per capita consumption of calories during the war was 2814—that is, only slightly less than the immediate prewar level of 2984 calories.[9] The height and weight of UK children and teenagers increased during the war years compared with the immediate prewar period. This improvement in nutrition was probably due to food rationing which resulted in better sharing of the available food among all social classes.

In Holland, food shortages, for some sections of the population, were severe at varying periods during the war years.[8] This may account for the 15% reduction in 1980–85 breast cancer mortality rates for 45–54 year old females who were children or teenagers during the war years.[7] However, this reduction is not statistically significant because breast cancer mortality rates in Holland did not rise for those women who were children and teenagers after the war years. However, other vital information was to emerge many years later from the Dutch wartime famine period.

As outlined in Chapter 7, nutritional experiences during childhood are the main factor determining the age at menarche. Other less influential factors include physical exercise, infections and possibly genetics. Early age at menarche is an established risk factor for breast cancer. While there is **anecdotal evidence**[2] that Norwegian children and teenagers probably did increase their physical exercise during the war years, it is most likely that the dietary restrictions were the most influential factor. While data is available that shows the gradual fall in menarcheal age from more than 17 years in the middle of the nineteenth century to a stable level of about 13.3 years for Norwegian women born after 1940, there is no detailed information about age at menarche relating to the war years.[6]

The Dutch famine 1944–45

Supplies of food during the war years in Holland, while far from generous, were adequate with one major exception—the famine of 1944–45.[10] In addition, it is known that, as for the UK, wartime rationing actually improved the diets of some previously disadvantaged Dutch children.

---

anecdotal evidence reports from personal experience

By mid-September 1944, the southern part of Holland, below the Rhine, had been liberated. The north remained occupied by the Germans, including the cities of Amsterdam, Rotterdam and The Hague. Dutch resistance workers organised a railroad strike in an effort to support the advance by British troops. These troops were to fight the famed and losing battle at the bridges crossing the Rhine river at Arnhem. This strike action prompted immediate retaliation by the Germans in the form of a complete embargo on the transport of food and fuel.

The situation rapidly became catastrophic as the hardest winter in 50 years descended. Ice blocked even canal traffic, exacerbating the German embargo on movements of supplies by road and rail. The great historic cities of Holland were worst affected, as they could not supplement their food supplies from the rural areas. Food rations decreased dramatically and for a period of seven months the only food available was bread and potatoes. By January 1945, food had dropped to 1000 calories per person per day (about half the normal consumption by a female) and had reached as low as 500 calories by April 1945. Food could not be brought into the famine area and the population could not travel to supplement supplies. Extra rations of food were allocated to pregnant women. The famine ceased abruptly with the liberation at the end of the war in May 1945.

While humans have suffered famine and pestilence throughout their evolution, the Dutch famine, together with the Norwegian wartime experience, is unique. This is largely because of the detailed documentation kept by the Dutch and Norwegian health and statistical authorities during and after the war. This action made possible an experiment on humans without scientific interference.

The first observation in Holland was that the age at menarche was delayed by eight months on average throughout the war years.[10] It is likely that the effect of caloric restriction on age at menarche was confined to girls who were already over ten years of age and expecting their first menstruation. The influence of any increase in exercise at this age for these Dutch girls is not known. This observation provides further supporting evidence for the relation between nutrition and age at menarche.

Mervyn Susser and Zena Stein now enter the story. Susser is a South African–American epidemiologist and a prolific writer, based in New York at Columbia University, where he now works as editor of the *American Journal of Public Health*. Stein, his long-time wife, work collaborator and friend, also from Columbia University, has a long background in the field of research into mental illness. They were getting nowhere with research aimed at giving socially deprived pregnant women extra food late in pregnancy with the aim of improving the infants' mental development, when they became aware of the Dutch famine and its possibilities for a natural experiment.

Together with Dutch colleagues, they began the laborious search through the detailed records that had kept track of all citizens during this time. Included in the data was information about pregnant women, including dates of birth and weights of their babies. With extraordinary insight they also tracked these babies and found most of them as adults. This was facilitated by the Dutch conscription of young men for military service. The military kept detailed psychological and physical records of 19-year-old males, all of which became available to the researchers. By linking the medical records, the dates and places of birth of Dutch soldiers, and intelligence tests 18 years later, the Susser–Stein team were able to make very detailed investigations. In addition, because of the Dutch tradition for record keeping, they were also able to search through hospital and school health records and to compile a lifetime history of the development of the babies who had been conceived and experienced intrauterine life during the famine.

The outcome of this natural study has been published intermittently since the 1970s and it is difficult to get an overview, but in summary the findings are as follows:

1 During the famine fertility declined.
2 Weights of mothers and birth weights of babies both declined below

expectations. However, birth weights declined only below a severe dietary threshold for the mother. In other words, the birth weight of the baby was maintained despite dietary restrictions on the mother until a particularly severe level of restriction was reached.

3 Famine affected the foetus in different ways depending on the gestational age (time since conception) of the foetus during nutritional deprivation of the mother.

The outcomes are extraordinary.[11,12] Nutritional deprivation during the first four months of pregnancy led to excess obesity of the offspring as 19-year-old adults, whereas deprivation during the last three months of pregnancy led to a reduction in obesity in the offspring as adults. These observations were first made in the male military recruits but have since been confirmed in adult Dutch females who were conceived during the famine.

It was shown that the famine had no deleterious effect on intellectual development but, unfortunately, there is an increased risk of schizophrenia in the now 50 year old infants conceived during the famine.

Finally, the observations on these Dutch citizens have been reproduced in experimental rats.[13]

 The implications of these experiences are that decreased nutrition during pregnancy has a potential effect on the offspring over decades, and that this effect is dependent on the degree of deprivation and the time it occurs during gestation.

Breast cancer has leftist tendencies

It has long been known that breast cancer in older women is up to 20% more common in the left breast.[14] This has been a consistent observation for more than 50 years and is therefore not simply due to

---

gestation growing period of the foetus

chance. However, the reason is completely obscure and, although Elizabeth also developed cancer in the left breast, no helpful conclusions can be drawn from this observation.

A wide range of reasons has been offered, but none confirmed. These include the greater size of the left as compared to the right breast, increased injury to the left breast, a protective effect of breastfeeding and genetics. The most plausible is the tendency for the left breast to be bigger than the right breast. Breast size in itself is probably not a risk factor for cancer, but Western women do have bigger breasts and higher risk of breast cancer than Asian women, and there may be an underlying cause. This may well be that larger breasts (i.e. left breasts) have a greater number of mammary gland cells and hence greater risk of breast cancer. **Also, there is a proven association between breast density and breast cancer, which appears to be more common in well fed Western women.**[15] Unfortunately, these observations have not helped in the search for the cause of breast cancer.

On the other hand, it has been clearly demonstrated that breast cancer is more common in left-handed than right-handed women.[16,17] This is yet another observation that defies belief, but potentially offers a clue. In an effort to explain these observations, studies have been carried out on schoolchildren to compare hand-use preference with their birth weight. It has been found that there is an association between high birth weight and left-hand preference in girls, and the reverse in boys.[18] The implications from these observations include a possible connection between nutrition and the hormones produced during pregnancy, between pregnancy hormones and brain development (which includes hand preference) in the foetus, and between all these influences and birth size, and subsequent increased risk of breast cancer.

At this stage this must all be speculative but, nevertheless, is supportive of the possibility that maternal nutrition influences future susceptibility to breast cancer.

Susser and Stein

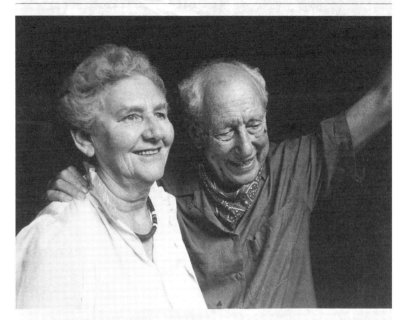

Zena Stein and Mervyn Susser

PERHAPS THE MOST INTERESTING DOCTORS in the field of epidemiology are Zena Stein and Mervyn Susser. Married in Durban, South Africa, in 1949, Mervyn and Zena's married life and working life were inextricably entwined. Throughout their entire careers, from a medical clinic in South Africa, to a medical school in England and then a public health school in the United States, this dynamic duo never worked or lived apart. Through their official work and private investigations they met with professional success on all three continents, Zena's more exuberant personality balancing Meryvn's quiet caution.

   Both ferociously intelligent, they embraced epidemiological study with a new and unique style of thinking. This was due largely to their concern with the effect of social and economic factors on public health—rather than simply looking at health in isolation. Each new case was tackled according to whether the results would make a difference to those most in need, be they poverty stricken, politically oppressed or simply uneducated and unable to help themselves.

Perhaps their most famous study was the investigation Mervyn and Zena led into the relationship between prenatal nutrition and mental development and competence later in life. The challenge lay in obtaining data on the weights of babies born to women who had suffered measurable malnutrition during the later stages of their pregnancy, and then finding follow-up data on these babies' mental ability later in life. The couple saw a possibility in the medical records of babies born to Dutch women during World War II.

For six months the northern part of Holland suffered from food shortages due to a Nazi blockade of food supplies, and children born after this period of hunger all showed a substantial fall in average birth weight. By linking the medical records, the dates and places of birth of Dutch soldiers, and intelligence tests 18 years later, the Susser–Stein team were able to make the most structured and conclusive investigations in the history of epidemiology.

Their comparisons indicated that malnutrition in pregnant mothers did not lead to reduced mental ability in their children. These results were contrary to the fashionable stance taken by most of the medical world at the time.

This exemplary couple are still alive and working today, as dedicated to their cause as they are to each other.

old and new ideas

False leads and negative outcomes

A breakthrough in the world of research is considered both as a mark of success to the person who made the discovery, and as a contribution to mankind. Pasteur, Florey and Salk are familiar names to schoolchildren throughout the world. Other, equally dedicated scientists can spend years searching for the cause of a health problem without ever making a new discovery. Not only is such work without the satisfaction of success, it is difficult to find an editor of a scientific journal who will publish negative findings. Editors have to sell their publications and readers are not attracted to reports showing that a particular pharmaceutical or surgical procedure does not work.

And so it has been with the search for the cause of breast cancer.

The most spectacular failure, if 'spectacular' can be used to describe a negative **outcome**, has been the search for the possible link between fats and breast cancer. Tannenbaum's 1942 finding that mice fed high-fat diets developed increased mammary tumours initiated the effort to find a similar link in humans. Early studies appeared to find such a link[1] but the methods used were flawed; it was not until major, expensive prospective trials were completed and reviewed more than 50 years later that reliable evidence became available showing that there was no link after all.[2] Even though this late

---

outcome the result of a research study

evidence appears to have completed the negative conclusion, new concepts have evolved which suggest that, while fat itself may not be the culprit, energy provided in the concentrated form of animal fats may well contribute to accelerated growth in the foetus and in childhood, and hence to increased cancers. We shall have to wait for the outcome.

There are many such negative findings in the field of breast cancer research. They include the influence of fibre, soy, tobacco, vitamins D and E, coffee and tea. Each of these has been explored, but with negative findings.

The nurses' toenails

The use of toenail clippings as a way of measuring levels of selenium in the body was mentioned earlier, but who would have believed that such clippings from 62 641 US nurses would provide evidence about breast cancer?

Arsenic, iron, copper, zinc and chromium have all at one stage been suspected of having some association with cancer. These are the so-called 'trace' metals, because they are present in the body in such small quantities, and have influenced cancer formation in animals and to a lesser extent in humans, either because they were present in too high levels, as in the case of arsenic, or too low levels, as for copper. So the exploration of an association in humans is justified. Scientists thought of the intriguing notion that the levels of these trace elements could be measured in humans without the need to take blood or remove tissue—through the simple collection of toenail clippings. And so, in 1982, participants in *The Nurses Health Study* in the United States were asked to provide toenail clippings from all ten toes (whether the clippings were identified toe by toe we do not know). The nurses were then followed for four years. No relationship could be found between the levels of any trace metal and breast cancer in any of the nurses.[3]

A breast cancer virus?

Perhaps the most important negative finding has been the failure to identify a virus as a cause of breast cancer. It has been known for many years that a virus was associated with mammary tumours in mice; indeed, many experimental mice are deliberately infected with the virus so as to provide what is called an 'experimental model' upon which other studies can be conducted.

Virus infections are known to be associated with some cancers in humans. The best known is Burkitt's lymphoma. This cancer of the lymphatic system (a drainage system with nodes in the armpits and groin) is caused by a virus spread in eastern and central Africa by mosquitoes. A more recently recognised viral cancer link is **cervical cancer** which is associated with infection by the common wart family of viruses. Accordingly, cervical cancer has become a sexually transmitted disease.

The negative link between such a virus and the possibility of breast cancer in humans is very fortunate and for a very good reason—AIDS.

There has been very little research into the historical beginnings of AIDS, and why should there be when the priority is to find a way of preventing AIDS in the future? Simply told, it seems likely that the AIDS virus has been present in some form for a great many years in African green monkeys. There may have been a mutation that made the AIDS virus so virulent. The conventional view is that it was such a virus that found its way into humans in central Africa and was then passed on to the United States via Haiti. In early 1998, evidence became available from studies on blood from central Africans that had been collected in 1959 and kept frozen for nearly 40 years which suggests that this theory may well be true.

However, an equally likely trail is that the green monkeys that carried the AIDS virus were captured in central Africa, sent to laboratories in the US and then returned as contaminated polio vaccines to the former Belgian Congo (now Republic of Congo). The early methods of preparation of polio vaccines were extremely

---

cervical cancer cancer of the cervix (neck of the womb)

crude. The polio virus was grown in green monkeys which were then killed and their kidneys, in which the virus concentrates, were ground up in a domestic-style meat mixer. The messy bits of monkey kidney were then filtered out through a muslin cloth, and the remainder injected into mice. The injection of the virus into mice is part of the *attenuation process* by which the virus is weakened and made safe for subsequent injection into human mothers and children. The serum from the mice is collected, put into phials, labelled and sold.

It is not widely known that at the time of the development of vaccines for polio during the 1950s there was a real fear that most of the world's children had been given a breast cancer virus.

Because the Sabin oral polio vaccine had been used in developed countries, including the former Soviet Union, new populations had to be sought for field trials of additional and different types of polio vaccine. Deals were done between the Wistar Institute of the US and the Belgian colonial authorities and trials began in the former Belgian Congo. After a latent period of perhaps 8–10 years there, the AIDS virus found its way back to the US, possibly through blood transfusions and the sexual activities of people moving between the Congo, Haiti and the US.

If we had known of the methods of preparation of the vaccine I doubt if many of us would have accepted vaccination with such literally open arms. Some scientists at the time expressed caution, because they know that such vaccines could carry unknown viruses. But the hysteria and concern about polio was so enormous that these objections were hardly heard, let alone acted upon. Fortunately, the mouse mammary tumour virus, which was almost certainly spread to humans through the vaccines, turned out to have no effect on human populations. But there is no doubt there could have been a disaster. Perhaps even more fortunate, there has been no link between the polio virus, the mouse mammary tumour virus and the AIDS virus.

Tobacco

From a public health perspective it is not relevant to determine whether tobacco smoking is a risk for breast cancer as the adverse associations of smoking are so great with respect to lung cancer and heart and other diseases. Therefore, the main interest in the role of tobacco smoking is to determine whether it can shed any light on the biology and cause of breast cancer. In brief, it does neither.

As we have come to expect with any aspect of breast cancer, considerable research effort has been expended on the search for a smoking relationship. There have been more than 20 substantial research studies into a possible relationship, but the results are indeterminate: some show that smoking increases, and others that it decreases, the risk of breast cancer. The probable reason for this smorgasbord of results lies in the differing methods and populations used in the studies. However, it can be concluded that there is no substantial contribution to breast cancer risk by tobacco smoking.[4,5]

This dogmatic and, to many, pleasing finding does not remove tobacco as a special risk factor for the health of women. On the contrary, there is solid evidence that women may be more sensitive than men to some of the harmful effects of smoking tobacco. The reason for this sex difference appears to be that tobacco smoke influences female metabolism (the chemistry of the body) by acting against the female sex hormones, oestrogens. Theoretically, such an anti-oestrogenic effect of tobacco smoking in women should reduce the risk of breast cancer, but it doesn't. Female tobacco smokers have an early menopause, a lowered risk of cancer of the endometrium (lining of the womb), a lowered risk of uterine fibroids and an increased risk of osteoporosis and of circulatory diseases such as coronary heart disease.[6] This increase in risk of heart disease is one-third higher than in men.[7]

Although such observations are not 'scientific', the anti-oestrogen effect on women can be readily seen in those who are heavy smokers. Such women tend to have a more masculine figure with less of a female body shape and a hair-line with a tendency to recede. They also tend to have collections of small capillary blood vessels on the face and the back of their hands.

Revolutionary ideas from an ancient land

For scientists seeking to solve the breast cancer problem, the 1980s was a decade of depression and failed hopes and expectations. Study after study produced negative findings. Nothing major had been found with respect to diet. Except for some minor protection by vitamin A, vitamins and minerals appeared to have no influence. No breast cancer virus had been found. There was a genetic factor but this could explain only about 5% of the problem.

The reproduction-related factors were well worked out but did not lead anywhere. The only progress was the confirmation that early-age exposure to hormones through early-age menarche increased the risk, but the main principles had been discovered 20 years before.

Workers tired of repeating studies that merely confirmed previous findings. A state of depression settled across the epidemiological world. Even the animal researchers had tired of the fight. They had shown again and again that high-fat diets increased the incidence of cancers of many types including breast cancer in rats and mice. But their work merely confirmed Tannenbaum's studies of the 1940s.

As the 1980s drew to a close, the possibility of preventing breast cancer had reached a dead end.

Inevitably, and very reasonably, the action moved to attempts at early diagnosis and treatment of breast cancer. These increasingly intense activities brought sound if slow rewards. After decades of little progress, work in Canada and New York began to show the value of mammography in the early diagnosis of breast cancer. The international women's movement began to lobby governments for financial support for mass mammography programs and, by the end of the decade, services were available in most developed countries.

At the same time progress was being made in the treatment of breast cancer. The most influential treatment was the new anti-oestrogen pharmaceuticals, the most effective being tamoxifen. These substances reduced the impact of oestrogens in women with established breast cancer. By 1995 survival rates for women diagnosed with breast cancer were improving by about 2% each year. These were fine achievements but, overall, breast cancer remained a formidable and seemingly insoluble problem.

The best brains in the medical world had reached an impasse.

Then, seemingly from nowhere, during 1988, two totally frustrated scientists offered some hope. They were de Waard from Holland and Trichopoulos from Greece. They were old friends and colleagues who had met at the regular scientific conferences that were organised to provide a forum for the discussion of common public health interests. For more than 15 years they had independently puzzled over the breast cancer problem. They also noted the negative outcomes of the many studies into diet and breast cancer that were so difficult to reconcile with international and experimental observations. During their discussions, the point was made that, while it was possible there may have been errors in the measurement of diets (people often underestimate how much they eat), it was also possible that the role of food as a cause of breast cancer was much more complex and subtle than had been assumed.

They began exactly the same journey that you have shared in this book. They first reviewed the known facts, then they reviewed the main theories of general cancer causation and finally they developed a revised theory or **hypothesis**. This simple but logical pattern of action and thinking led them to the view that the key to breast cancer was possibly the consumption of 'energy-rich' diets during childhood and adolescence which exerted a step-by-step effect through hormones, of which oestrogen played a major part. In late 1988 they published their thoughts in the *International Journal of Cancer*.[8]

---

hypothesis idea based on limited evidence, awaiting proof

For a scientist there is nothing worse than silence; even a dissenting voice is better than nothing. But there was no reaction from the scientific community to the publication of the unifying theory by de Waard and Trichopoulos. Perhaps no one had read the article. Perhaps colleagues were unimpressed but too kind to say so.

But, unknown to the authors, their ideas had been read and taken seriously by two rather obscure epidemiologists working in Milan. Franco Berrino and Gemma Gatta had been interested in the problem of breast cancer for some time for the very good reason that every year increasing numbers of Italian women were contracting the disease. They noted that women who had migrated as adults from the south to the north of Italy, after World War II, had much less breast cancer than their daughters who had migrated at the same time.[9] While the researchers did not have details of the diets consumed by these internal Italian migrants, they knew that the people of the south had a much lower intake of proteins and fats than the people of the north. These observations were exactly as hypothesised by de Waard and Trichopoulos. So the Italians wrote a letter to the same journal, outlining this information. This rekindled interest in the view that it was diet in young people and not in adults that was the main influence on subsequent risk of breast cancer.

But interest and opinions are insufficient; much more proof was needed. It was to be nearly 10 years before these early observations were confirmed by large studies in Italy.[10]

Some say the best export from Greece is the people. Names such as Pete Sampras and Mark Philippoussis, the tennis stars of Greek origin, suggest there may be some truth in this. One name you won't be as familiar with is that of Dimitrios Trichopoulos, a man who is as influential in the modern world of epidemiology as were the famed Greek heroes of the ancient world.

In preparation for this book, I wrote to Dimitrios Trichopoulos to try to obtain some details about his life and background. Given his obvious intellectual stature, I thought he might have millennia-old family connections to the great Greek thinkers of the past. He may well

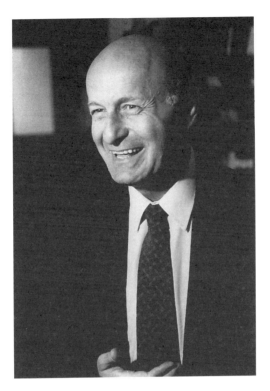

Dimitrios Trichopoulos, one of the most influential Greek scientists since Archimedes and Aristotle. He was among the first to recognise the risks associated with passive tobacco smoking. In 1990 he developed the hypothesis that prenatal influences, including maternal nutrition, influenced subsequent risk of breast cancer in female offspring. This has led to an intense and rewarding international research effort.

have such famous genes coursing through his veins, but if so he is not going to tell anyone. He responded to my letter in one sentence: 'My life is so exceedingly simple that it can be summarized in … essentially one sentence: working and travelling for work.'

Trichopoulos had been doing routine research work in Athens and Boston during the 1980s and was able to make modest contributions to knowledge about diet and breast cancer when, together with F de Waard, he published the quiet paper suggesting that diets consumed by children may be the missing breast cancer link. As we noted, this paper and these ideas caused hardly a comment. Perhaps this was because the paper appeared in the rather obscure *International Journal of Cancer*, or perhaps it was because there seemed to be nothing remarkable about their ideas—Cole and MacMahon had espoused the same principles nearly 20 years before—or perhaps it was because both de Waard and Trichopoulos came from what were regarded by some as lesser centres of learning, de Waard from Utrecht and Trichopoulos from Athens. However, regardless of their origins, this pair of epidemiologists were scholars of the highest order. De Waard had led the scientific world with his descriptions of the natural history of breast cancer and in 1981 Trichopoulos had been among the first to recognise that passive smoking was associated with lung cancer. Nearly a decade on, the de Waard and Trichopoulos publication is worth revisiting.[8]

From the basis of 15 years' work in the field of breast cancer epidemiological research, de Waard and Trichopoulos brought together a number of well established facts. Their first concept was to think of the development of breast cancer as a series of steps on the way to the development of full **malignancy**. They believed these steps began before puberty and continued during adolescence. They noted the experimental work in mice and rats showing early growths in mammary glands that were not malignant. They regarded these growths as the forerunners of hormone-induced cancers and were aware of observations in humans that were similar to those of the cells in the experimental animals. In addition, they noted the patterns of breast cancer in migrants, the international variation in breast cancer, and the increases in breast cancer that were taking place in Japan. They noted the increased risk associated with early menarche and tallness, and the increased sensitivity to malignant change from exposure to radiation during early childhood and the peripubertal period. They also noted the high oestrogen levels that occur in girls who have an early menarche. They also took into account other factors such as the protection from breast cancer by early age at first full-term pregnancy. Finally, they hypothesised that the influence of

---

malignancy a cancer with the potential for uncontrollable growth and spread

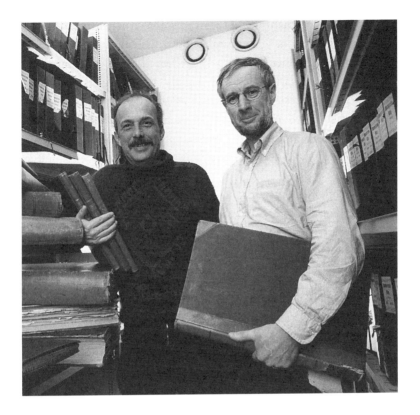

Hans-Olaf Adami and Anders Ekbom, leaders of a research team from Sweden, who provided the first evidence in humans that events during pregnancy could influence the risk of subsequent breast cancer in daughters more than 50 years later.

excess weight came from the production of oestrogens from the excess fat.

These observations have been considered in some detail earlier in this book. The key step by Trichopoulos and de Waard was to put together these seemingly disparate facts and to develop a coherent overview.

In essence, they proposed that early menarche and tall body height are associated with but do not cause the formation of breast lesions that have increased cancer potential, and that these phenomena are produced by early maturing of the ovaries as a response to an energy-rich diet in childhood. They postulated that such nutrition was rich in an energy sense, rather than a specific effect of fat or other nutrients accelerating the ovarian ripening. Finally, they suggested that late menopause and obesity act much later as cancer enhancers. They also made predictions about several events, including the possible decrease in breast cancer among those who experienced food deprivation during World War II—as we know, this prediction has been found to be accurate.

Ever modest, de Waard and Trichopoulos emphasise that these ideas were not new, but merely offered a rewritten version of the work of previous scientists. To a substantial extent this is so, but they added a previously missing emphasis on the influence of diet *at a young age* and the time sequence of events.

However, there was a major flaw in their concept, which any informed person can calculate on the back of an envelope: that is, the concept accounts for only about 150% of the increased risk of breast cancer in Western as compared with Asian women, whereas there needs to be a hypothesis that accounts for the actual 400–600% difference in risk.

Trichopoulos' activities were to be a mere prelude to his next contribution. Two years later, in 1990, he hypothesised in the *Lancet* (a century-old British-based medical journal) that breast cancer was initiated in the foetus![11]

But a hypothesis is just that, a hypothesis. It is not proof. But Trichopoulos was to use his diplomatic skills to encourage others to seek to prove his ideas. His influence spread to a remarkable Swedish group led by Hans-Olaf Adami and Anders Ekbom, and to the already substantial Harvard group led by the elders of the breast cancer epidemiological game, Frank Speizer, Walter Willett, David Hunter and, latterly, Graham Colditz and Karin Michels. The search for proof of this new theory was now on in earnest.

But before considering this search for proof, a summary of Trichopoulos' second hypothesis is necessary.

The Trichopoulos hypothesis on prenatal influences

Trichopoulos' first realisation was that his previous hypothesis, which had been developed in collaboration with de Waard, did not, as we observed above, account for the marked international differences in incidence of breast cancer. Then, as for all hypotheses, he again began with a review of the accepted facts and observations.[11] We have already given some consideration to many of these facts and they do not need to be repeated. However, he reviewed some factors that we have not considered. These are:

1 Chemicals can cause **prenatal** (before birth) cancer in some animals.
2 Intrauterine exposure of the foetus to radiation can cause leukaemia and other tumours in children.
3 Artificial oestrogens taken during pregnancy can cause vaginal cancers in daughters.
4 Exposure to atom bomb radiation in childhood resulted in increased cancers, including breast cancers, at the normal adult age for such cancers; that is, there was a long latent period between exposure and the cancer.
5 High intrauterine exposure to natural oestrogens increases testicular and ovarian cancers.

Based on these observations, Trichopoulos made the seemingly simple suggestion that increased concentrations of oestrogens in pregnancy (possibly with increased concentrations of other pregnancy hormones) increase the probability of daughters getting breast cancer by creating a 'fertile soil' for subsequent cancer initiation.

In making this hypothesis he made four assumptions:

1 Oestrogens are important factors for breast cancer.
2 Factors that increase cancer after birth also do so prenatally.
3 Oestrogen concentrations are ten times higher than normal during pregnancy.

---

prenatal before birth

4   Oestrogen concentrations during pregnancy vary widely between individual women.

Finally, he noted a range of studies that had been done or needed to be done in order to prove his theories. One of the more important of these was already known and was later to be of great relevance to the breast cancer story. This was the discovery by Petridou and his colleagues in Athens (which included Trichopoulos) that pregnancy oestrogens are important determinants of birth weight.[12]

It was to be Adami and Ekbom's Swedish group who were largely able to confirm, by indirect observations, Trichopoulos' theories. They were able to do so primarily because of the culture of Sweden itself. The Swedes keep records of a rather personal and very detailed nature about everybody and everything, to a degree that would be regarded as a severe invasion of privacy by Americans, and certainly by Australians. From birth each individual is given a unique number which is kept for life. This number allows for the follow-up in an accurate way of details of birth weight, marriage, age at first birth and, of course, sickness and death. These were the very facts that Dimitrios Trichopoulos had foreshadowed as being necessary to prove his theories.

But not only culture was needed. Talent, hard work and interest were necessary and came from Hans-Olaf Adami, Anders Ekbom and colleagues, supported by Dimitrios Trichopoulos himself. By 1992 they had showed indirectly that concentrations of oestrogens during pregnancy were related to subsequent breast cancer risk.[13] This was done by noting that women who were large as babies were at greater risk of breast cancer, and those women who had an illness known as **pre-eclampsia,** or toxaemia of pregnancy (a condition characterised by high blood pressure followed by convulsions and death if not successfully treated), were at less risk of breast cancer. As noted above, another Greek group, led by Petridou and colleagues, had found that women with high oestrogens during pregnancy had larger than average babies. The size of the baby is not a risk factor—

pre-eclampsia toxaemia of pregnancy

it is a surrogate indicator of complex underlying processes probably associated with hormone chemistry and growth.

The Swedish group not only developed evidence, they began to develop their own theories. These included the suggestion that, while oestrogens are not directly responsible for cancer initiation, they do enhance the reproduction of cells (i.e. growth) and that the higher rate of cell production increases the likelihood of mistakes, leading to genetic changes and ultimately to cancer.

While these Swedish activities were taking place, a US group from Boston, led by Thomas Sandson, made the intriguing discovery that women with breast cancer often had different brain symmetry from women without breast cancer.[14] The brain develops in response to micronutrients and micro-hormones during early foetal life, and any upset in these hormone levels can lead to different development. This study was made possible by the development of sophisticated computerised X-ray examinations that give a three-dimensional picture of the brain. Such an observation in women with breast cancer indicates changes in the 'normal' intrauterine hormonal environment, again as had been predicted by Trichopoulos.

Since that time, studies involving many thousands of women have confirmed the probable link between birth weight and breast cancer.[15,16] However, Ekbom and colleagues, plus Trichopoulos of course, in a very recent expansion of their earlier study that included more than 1000 Swedish women with breast cancer did not find an association between birth weight and breast cancer.[17] But they did confirm a range of fascinating facts.

Breast cancer risk was increased among those who as infants had been twins (dizygotic, i.e. not identical), severely premature, had neonatal jaundice (yellow pigmentation of the skin after birth) and whose mothers were older. All these conditions are associated with higher than normal pregnancy oestrogen levels. This was in contrast to the markedly reduced risk of breast cancer found in women whose mothers had pregnancy pre-eclampsia (also known as toxaemia characterised by high blood pressure and convulsions) and lower than normal pregnancy oestrogen levels.

The search for additional evidence is now under way on a worldwide basis. The early evidence showing that **dizygotic twins** who experience high levels of maternal oestrogens during prenatal life and subsequently experience significantly increased risk of breast cancer has been confirmed in several studies, including a large British study involving 500 twins with breast cancer.[18] The current interest in twins has rekindled earlier interest in this issue. In the mid-1950s German scientists demonstrated that identical twins (i.e. those with the same genetic material) had very different lifetime experiences with cancer. The twin who was heavier at birth was much more likely to develop a range of cancers. These findings were confirmed by Richard Osborne and Frances De George working in the United States.[19] The obvious conclusion is that environmental influences, mainly during pregnancy, were more influential on subsequent cancer development than genetic influences.

In addition, there appears to be a direct relationship between birth weight and infant mammary gland development at birth.[20] It is a common observation to see swollen breasts and a milk-like excretion from the breasts of large infants.

Despite Ekbom's negative finding, the overall findings are compatible with observations of populations which show that breast cancer is less common in Asian Americans than in Caucasian American women and that they have, on average, smaller infants.[21]

We have gathered data from countries of both low and high risk of breast cancer which shows that, in low-risk countries, the consumption of calories is much less, and also the average birth weight is less than in high-risk countries. These observations are shown in Table 10.1. However, such observations are subject to error and must be treated with caution.

---

dizygotic twins non-identical twins

Table 10.1 Associations between average infant birth weight, national per capita food consumption at time of birth, and annual breast cancer mortality per 100 000 females aged 35–54 years for selected countries
This information shows that there is an association between average size of babies in a given population and subsequent risk of breast cancer. In addition it is likely that those mothers who gave birth to small babies consumed less energy than those mothers who gave birth to large babies. The inference is that rich diets consumed during pregnancy lead to increased growth of babies, who are at subsequent increased risk of breast cancer. However, these conclusions need additional confirmation.

Country	Infant birth weight for various years, 1945/1965	Calories per capita per day, various years, 1945–1965	Breast cancer mortality, various years, 1991/1994	
			Age 35–44	Age 45–54
China	3100	1500	urban 4.0	13.4
			rural 6.9	12.0
Hong Kong	3100	2500	7.7	22.3
Japan	3070	1900	9.5	20.0
West Germany	3270	2890	17.6	48.0
Switzerland	3290	3100	13.9	44.3
United States	3320	3090	16.1	42.6
Poland	3350	3300	13.6	38.2
United Kingdom	3350	3250	19.2	54.2
Czechoslovakia	3350	3000	15.1	44.9
Israel	3200	3400	19.9	52.7

Countries selected because of availability of data. Mortality data is for Germany as a whole. *Sources:* 1. Meredith HV. Body Weight at birth of viable human infants: a worldwide comparative treatise. Human Biol. 1970; 42: 217–64. 2. World Health Statistics Annual 1995, WHO Geneva 1996. 3. Food Supply-Time Series. Food and Agriculture Organisation, Rome. Food Balance Sheets, Food and Agriculture Organisation, Rome, 1996.

Elizabeth Sutherland fits into this risk profile. Her mother conscientiously ate huge amounts of milk, cheese and meat during her pregnancy with Elizabeth. She then gave birth to a large baby, Elizabeth. In turn, this baby was also fed a rich diet, which led to early menarche. As a young adult, Elizabeth maintained what to her was her normal diet, plenty of 'wholesome' meat, milk, cheese and vegetables, plus the new-for-Australia, American-style takeaways

provided by McDonald's and Kentucky Fried Chicken. She put on
weight during her 'pregnant period', which seemed natural to her. In
summary, Elizabeth behaved in exactly the normal way for a middle-
class Australian.

There are animal experiments on mice and rats which show that, if mothers are fed high-fat diets, the risk of mammary tumours in daughters is increased.[22-24] This is similar to the link between human maternal diets and birth weights that was shown so dramatically by the Dutch famine natural experiment.[25] It will be recalled that this showed nutrition deprivation influenced obesity in adult offspring depending on the timing during pregnancy of the deprivation. Nutrition deprivation during the first half of pregnancy led to adult obesity, but similar deprivation during the last three months of pregnancy led to reduced rates of adult obesity in offspring. The implication of these findings is that nutritional experiences of the mother during different periods of her pregnancy lead to different but lifelong influences on offspring.

It is difficult to know what influence these experimental studies on the effects of diet during pregnancy and mammary cancers in offspring of rats had on Dimitrios Trichopoulos, as he does not refer to the work of Boeryd and colleagues who had published their findings in 1986, well before his 1990 hypothesis. While experiments in animals are not necessarily paralleled in humans, when the experiences are the same the evidence becomes very strong that similar events are happening.

Ordinary citizens could not care less which particular scientist was the first to offer new theories or the first to make a new discovery. However, for scientists, the issue of primacy—that is, to be the first—is as important as life itself. This is because recognition by peers, funding authorities and the history of science is greatly influenced by being the first. Even such angelic and historic figures as Charles Darwin were stimulated to be the first to publish by competitors. In Darwin's case this was Alfred

Wallace, who wrote to Darwin outlining his own observations about the origins of species. Darwin was worried about the potential public backlash that might be set off by his revolutionary ideas and it was only the threat of loss of primacy that influenced him to publish his work immediately.

Already, scientists such as Van Assche from Belgium are claiming to have 'published the first article on the long-term consequences of an abnormal intrauterine environment'.[26] Van Assche has made a sound contribution to this field but the concept that events during pregnancy influence subsequent health of the offspring goes back to at least the 1930s, when the origin of diabetes was being explored. The earliest work that links breast cancer to the size of infants appears to be that of Lev Berstein and his colleague EK Hint, who published their findings in 1970. They showed that the parents of large babies were at twice the risk of breast cancer than parents of small babies.[27] Berstein has done most of his work in St Petersburg and nearly all his publications have been in Russian; however unfair it may be, his work is therefore not widely known. As with much new knowledge, scientists tend to be influenced both consciously and unconsciously by preceding work; inevitably, Trichopoulos would have been influenced by the emerging knowledge of links between a variety of cancers and prenatal events. However, Trichopoulos put the relevant facts together and formed the coherent theory that has stimulated so much interest, and much of the credit is deservedly his.

To complicate the picture further, recent evidence has emerged that different types of fat may alter the chemistry of the body in different ways.[28] This was discussed earlier in the context of lifelong patterns of nutrition, in the chapters on diet and breast cancer. This evidence is that monounsaturated fats, as found in olive oil, may reduce breast cancer risk and that polyunsaturated fats, as found in vegetable margarines, but not saturated fats, as found in meats and dairy products, may increase breast cancer risk. The recent findings that consumption of high polyunsaturated fats by pregnant rats increases

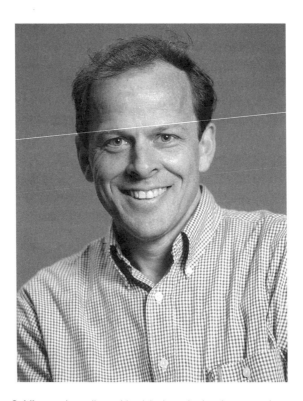

Graham Colditz, an Australian epidemiologist, who has been a major contributor to *The Nurses Health Study* since 1981. In recent years he has been encouraging the development of breast cancer prevention strategies in young people. A prolific author, he has published scientific articles on many issues accociated with breast cancer.

mammary cancer in female offspring is in sympathy with this additional finding.[24]

The nutritional status of mothers during pregnancy also influences the number of non-identical twins that are born. It has no influence on the number of identical twins. This is known from World War II experiences.[29] Those western European countries that suffered nutritional deprivation during the war, Norway, Holland and France, all experienced a fall in the proportion of non-identical twins. This has been attributed to the influence of nutrition during pregnancy on hormone metabolism and the lowered production of double ovulations, but not on divided fertilised ova that lead to identical twins. These findings provide added evidence for a powerful influence of nutrition during pregnancy on hormone metabolism.

Collectively, the results of these various studies and observations of populations are compatible with **perinatal** factors being associated with breast cancer risk in the offspring. The evidence that it is pregnancy oestrogen levels alone is not strong and it would be expected that the underlying mechanisms are far more complex than a single hormone.

For example, **growth hormones** are likely to be influential. Such hormones are necessary for the growth of most tissues including the milk ducts in the breast (i.e. the most common sites of breast cancer). It has recently been discovered that high levels of growth hormones circulating in the blood of premenopausal women are associated with a doubling of the risk of breast cancer.[30] Although additional evidence is needed, there is a probable link between diet and growth hormones. Energy-restricted diets that decrease growth hormones also decrease the incidence of breast cancer in rats.[31]

In addition, there are associations between growth hormone levels in the body and birth weight and height, which are in turn associated with breast cancer risk.

Thus we have good knowledge about the likely basic risk factors for breast cancer, but do not always have direct proof, nor do we have detailed knowledge of the mechanisms of cancer formation. There is also another possibility—is the problem multi-generational? Are grandmothers also responsible for breast cancer?

There is one more problem. The concept that events during prenatal life could be involved with the development of cancer four, five or six decades later is so extraordinary that it is difficult to accept for those unfamiliar with the evidence. The first reaction is simply one of disbelief: 'There go those crazy scientists again.' But it is possible. The evidence is sound (though short of an accepted high level of scientific proof) and it is the best chance we have so far of seeking to develop effective primary prevention strategies.

---

perinatal around the time of birth
growth hormone a chemical substance carried in the blood which influences the growth of most tissues of the body

In addition to this work on the foetus and breast cancer, there have been parallel developments in knowledge about the foetus and a range of other diseases, including cardiovascular disease (coronary heart disease and stroke) and diabetes; it has been demonstrated that very low birth weights are associated with increased cardiovascular disease.[32] There is also limited evidence showing that very low birth weights may be associated with lower than normal intellectual capacity during adulthood.[33] It will be recalled that such an observation was considered but not made in the Dutch famine studies. This new knowledge adds to the body of evidence in support of the concept that events during prenatal life can have a lifelong impact.

Breast cancer risks from grandmothers

Is breast cancer risk intergenerational?

Grandmothers make an obvious genetic contribution to breast cancer risk in their grand-daughters, but do they also make an additional contribution related to diet and birth weight?

As we have discussed, considerable evidence has accumulated to confirm indirectly Trichopoulos' hypothesis that maternal diets and pregnancy hormones might be important determinants of breast cancer risk in daughters.[11,34]

Studies of females who migrate from low- to high-risk breast cancer countries show that it takes two generations for the risk of breast cancer to reach that of the host population.[35,36] This delay has been attributed to the retention of traditional diets. However, such migrants experience rapid increases in risk of cancer of the colon and reach rates similar to those of the host population within one generation. Many migrants and their children retain traditional patterns of food consumption, but substantially increase consumption of sugars, meats and animal fats and traditional festival foods quickly become daily diets.[37,38]

There is no doubt about the biological feasibility of intergenerational **carcinogenic** (cancer-initiating) influences. The most dramatic instance of such influence is vaginal cancer in the daughters of mothers who have consumed artificial oestrogens.[39] Examples of more subtle influences are the increased risk of childhood leukaemia,[40] and a variety of other cancers in those who were large babies.[41]

Recently, Skjaerven and colleagues[42] showed decisively that the weight of a baby is strongly associated with the baby's mother's birth weight and, one could imply, the birth weight of the baby's grandmother.

The evidence that the average size of newborn babies in a given population depends largely on the nutritional experiences of the mother is compelling—particularly the evidence, discussed earlier, from the Dutch famine. Detailed documentation showed that nutritional deprivation not only influenced the size of the baby but had very different influences according to the **gestation** of the foetus at the time of deprivation.[43]

There is an intriguing additional outcome from the Dutch famine that has only just begun to emerge—namely, that the influence of nutrition on the foetus may cross generations. Lumey and a group of colleagues in Amsterdam have been studying the offspring of the offspring of the babies conceived during the famine and have found they are also of smaller birth weight than average.[44] This finding has ominous implications with respect to breast cancer, because rapid preventive action will be extremely difficult if the causes are intergenerational.

Intergenerational influences on birth weight, and therefore possibly breast cancer, include genetics, diet and energy expenditure, and tobacco smoking. The most influential is almost certainly diet.[45,46] This is because:

- few women smoke in populations at low risk of breast cancer such as Japan and China, and
- genetics influences only about 5% of women with breast cancer.

---

carcinogenic cancer-initiating
gestation stage of development of pregnancy and foetus

The degree of influence of genetics on birth size is debatable. Some studies of fathers and of twins suggest the influence may be considerable, but this is in contrast to other studies which suggest that genetics is a negligible influence on birth size and that socioeconomic factors, in particular diet, are dominant.[46]

Among Western women, particularly those of high socioeconomic status, the risk of breast cancer has been high for most of the twentieth century. Such women have had ready access to ample food and have not had to exercise strenuously during pregnancy. As a consequence they have had, on average, large babies who, in turn, have become mothers who were also likely to have large babies. Such babies were probably, as adults, at increased risk of breast cancer. It seems possible that grandmothers are an 'old' risk of breast cancer.

In formal terms, the evidence is suggestive, but incomplete, that breast cancer has intergenerational origins.

It is at least arguable that Elizabeth's mother and her mother's mother also contributed to her breast cancer. In part, this may have been genetic, but it was possibly due to the intergenerational effects of diet. Each successive mother had sufficient economic resources to give them access to rich food during their pregnancy. Each had a rather large baby which tended also to have large babies, and large babies are an indicator of growth and production of high levels of pregnancy hormones, which appear to enhance the subsequent risk of breast cancer.

---

so what
do we know?

If you have struggled this far and feel overburdened with facts, figures and sophisticated technical terms, you are in very good company. After decades of research and the publication of thousands of scientific papers on the problem of breast cancer, by the 1990s the world's leading scientists had also become dismayed at the lack of progress, although the basic epidemiological facts about breast cancer were well established.

As a reminder, these facts are:

1 Breast cancer occurs almost entirely in females.
2 While most deaths due to breast cancer occur in old age, one in four deaths occurs before the age of 50 years.
3 Breast cancer is up to six times more common in Western countries but, when Asian women migrate to the West, within two generations they experience a similar risk to the indigenous population of the host country.
4 Breast cancer appears to run in families—that is, it has a genetic component.
5 Early age at menarche is associated with increased risk.
6 Early-age first full-term pregnancy reduces risk, and late-age first full-term pregnancy increases risk. Never to have been pregnant increases the risk.
7 Late-age menopause increases risk.

8 Being overweight after menopause may increase risk.

9 To be tall increases risk.

10 To be of high social status increases risk.

11 To drink alcohol increases risk.

12 The incidence of breast cancer is increasing in developing countries.

13 National per capita energy, protein and fat consumption is associated with breast cancer risk.

14 Breast cancer is not caused by a virus, or chemicals, but increases many years after irradiation of young females by atom bombs, X-rays or other forms of radiation.

Poor Elizabeth Sutherland—some 90% of these facts or risks applied to her. She was a relatively young Western female of high social status, she was fed an energy-rich diet (according to the guidelines for her day) as a child and teenager, she was breastfed but only for a few months, her menarche was early and she drank the (then) fashionable two glasses of wine each evening. From a breast cancer perspective, the only protection she had was her relatively early first baby. She wasn't to know, but being the daughter and grand-daughter of women with an almost identical background had probably compounded her risk.

This list is so complex and, seemingly, so without reason that it is difficult to remember, let alone try to understand. Hence the need for the development of some insightful **hypotheses**. Apart from Tannenbaum's observations that high-fat diets fed to mice increased mammary tumours and the related hypothesis that similar diets fed to humans would cause breast cancer, the first comprehensive theories (*hypothesis* and *theory* mean the same thing, i.e. ideas based on limited evidence that need to be proven) were developed in 1969 by Philip Cole and Brian MacMahon, who had undertaken

---

hypothesis idea based on limited evidence, awaiting proof

extensive epidemiological work at the Harvard School of Public Health. They **postulated** (i.e. put forward the idea) that breast cancer may be initiated at an early age and then promoted by the sex hormone oestrogen.[1] They based their ideas on three known features of the disease:

1 the reduction in breast cancer in women who have their ovaries surgically removed
2 the lifetime reduction in breast cancer among women who have an early age pregnancy
3 the low incidence of breast cancer in Asian and African populations.

The first observation supports the belief that ovarian hormones (i.e. oestrogens) play a major role in human breast cancer. The second observation supports the belief that early reproductive experiences are influential in the initiation or promotion of breast cancer. This view is supported by the retention of the low incidence of breast cancer, characteristic of Japan, by Japanese migrants and their daughters to the US, plus the protective effect of early full-term pregnancy. The third observation is compatible with the finding that some components of oestrogen are associated with increased cancer activity and that other components inhibit cancer activity. These inhibitory components have been found at higher levels in Chinese woman as compared with Caucasian women. Cole and MacMahon were of the view that the number of years between puberty and first pregnancy may be a crucial determinant of a woman's lifetime breast cancer risk.

The significance of these hypotheses was to be the reordering of research priorities from older to younger women. This is a radical change: until the time of the Cole–MacMahon hypothesis, the orthodox view was that cancers were predominantly a problem associated with ageing, and that latent periods of decades between the initiation and the appearance of a clinical cancer were inconceivable.

While the link between age at menarche and risk of breast cancer had long been recognised, researchers slowly began to give attention

---

postulate put forward an idea

to the determinants—that is, the causes of the age at menarche. This was to take more than two decades to resolve.

Further, few had taken the 'duck principle' seriously. The central tenet of the duck principle is that if you are sitting by a lake and you see a bird about the size of a grown chicken, it has feathers and a bill, it swims with the help of webbed feet and looks like a duck, it is highly probable that it is a duck. In the case of breast cancer, there is an obvious and repeatedly observed association between the high rates of breast cancer and consumption of energy-rich foods in given populations. Applying the duck principle leads to the obvious conclusion that food consumption patterns must in some way be associated with breast cancer. However, leading scientists, including members of the famed Harvard University group, insisted that the duck principle did not apply because of the lack of reliability of the international data.[2] Their views were supported by the lack of evidence of an association between high fat consumption during adult life and breast cancer.

Over the years many scientists have developed theoretical concepts about the causative mechanisms of breast cancer. The ideas of Cole and MacMahon led to interest in factors that operate in young people; de Waard and Trichopoulos developed a unified theory that brought the fragmented observations together and led to the concept of a step-by-step development of breast cancer over decades; and Trichopoulos developed the prenatal concept of the causation of breast cancer which led to the explosion of research into the influences of the pregnant environment on breast cancer. So theories are not simply the musings of clever people—they can lead to decisive action.

The Swedish contribution

A group of Swedish scientists, headed by Hans-Olaf Adami and in collaboration with Dimitrios Trichopoulos, has prepared the most up-to-date review of the known evidence and developed a detailed theoretical outline of the possible mechanics behind the development of breast cancer. This work was published in *Mutation Research*, a leading scientific journal in the world of genetic science but almost completely unknown elsewhere.[3] This is a pity because this contribution deserves to be more widely known. The title of the paper, 'The aetiology and pathogenesis of human breast cancer', gives some idea of the problem of converting their ideas into plain English. We have prepared a summary of their ideas to help you follow their thoughts.

Environmental factors, in a broad sense, play a dominant role in the cause of human breast cancer (as distinct from mouse mammary cancers which can be caused by a virus). This opinion was based initially on the difference in the incidence of breast cancer between people in different countries. Theoretically, such differences between populations and ethnic groups might be due to genetic differences rather than the environment. However, studies of migrants, mainly but not only from Japan, a low-risk population for breast cancer, to the United States clearly showed that rates of breast cancer approached the high rates in the US by the third generation. This excluded the possibility that these differences in breast cancer risk have exclusively a genetic basis. However, this view does not exclude important environmental/genetic interactions. Nor does it deny that genetic traits may be sufficient causes in their own right for about 5% of total breast cancer.

Also, any causal theory must accommodate the fact that breast cancer is at least 100 times more common in women than men.

The established association between breast cancer and age at menarche and at menopause supports the conclusion that production of hormones from the ovaries is essential for the development of most breast cancers. It has also been shown beyond doubt that the effect of pregnancy on the breast depends on the age at which the pregnancy takes place. The earlier the first full-term pregnancy the more protection against breast cancer.

It is likely that some aspects of diet are important as causes of breast cancer, despite the evidence that dietary fat in adult life is not at all associated, or at most weakly associated, with breast cancer risk. This observation about dietary fat in adult life is compatible with the possibility that fat consumption, or energy intake, and expenditure (mainly through exercise) early in life is an important determinant of breast cancer risk.

The hypothesis that breast cancer may originate in the uterus was, as we have discussed, developed by Trichopoulos. He suggested that high levels of pregnancy hormones, particularly but not only oestrogens, might create a 'fertile soil' for the establishment or initiation of subsequent cancer. The studies that we have considered have given indirect support for this concept.

It has been argued that the differences in breast cancer risk between populations could be explained by different reproductive experiences, in particular the younger age of first birth in developing countries at low risk of breast cancer. However, detailed examination of trends has shown that this is a far from adequate explanation for the fivefold difference between countries.

The theory that breast cancer risk is already programmed in the uterus would be supported if some differences in the structure of the breasts of newborn babies could be found. This has been found by the studies of Anbazhagan who showed that newborn babies had breasts at widely varying stages of development. Some had many milk-producing lobules, others had none. These lobules continue to develop until they become fully mature, or specialised, during post-pregnancy lactation. The rate of cell multiplication is greater in the non-specialised, or immature, lobules than in the specialised mature lobules. This high rate of cell turnover, or multiplication, is believed to be associated with an increased likelihood of genetic errors that could lead to loss of growth control—that is, cancer. Thus, the earlier puberty starts and the later a first full-term pregnancy takes place the greater the risk.

A more difficult issue is to identify which factors determine these structural developments in the newborn baby, and at a later age in pubertal and adult breasts. The prime candidates are ovarian hormones, although it is likely that other hormones and growth-related chemicals such as insulin play a role. The development of full malignant transformation of a normal cell is likely to be enhanced by the continued exposure to hormones.

The Swedish group has not considered the relationship between food consumption patterns and breast cancer risk. This has been the province of a range of other workers who have shown that food consumption patterns are probable influences on hormone production in females.[4-6]

'Strength of the evidence' explained

When evaluating the *strength of the evidence* relating to causes of cancer it is appropriate to use standard terms. These standard words and phrases have been developed and adopted by the International Agency for Research on Cancer. This organisation, with headquarters based in Lyons, France, is part of the World Health Organisation.

The term 'sufficient evidence' is used when direct evidence is available; the term 'limited evidence' is used when the evidence is indirect. *Direct evidence* refers to first-hand observation; *indirect evidence* refers to circumstantial observations. An example of a direct observation is the actual measurement of food eaten by children, who are then followed up and the precise age at menarche observed and recorded. This is in contrast to indirect evidence where adult women are asked to recall details of their diets as children and to remember their age at menarche. Direct evidence is obviously more reliable.

Of importance to those who are not familiar with biomedical terminology is use of the word 'significant'. In biomedical journals, use of the term 'significant' implies that the results of research are statistically significant—that is, the results can be relied on to have a 95% chance of being accurate or true. In the biomedical field (which includes studies of cancer, infections and chemistry in humans and animals) this approach is usually expressed as a **confidence interval** (CI). A 95% CI means there is a 95% chance that the results of a research study are accurate or true between a range of results. For example, the results of the meta-analyses (reviews of all the data from a collection of studies considering the same issues) that consider the possible relationship between alcohol consumption and breast cancer risk indicate there is a 95% likelihood or confidence interval that it is true or accurate that women who consume two standard alcoholic drinks per day have between 1.4 and 2.2 times increased risk of breast cancer, compared with women who do not consume any alcohol.

Unfortunately, even if such results are assessed by the researchers and editors of scientific journals as being 'significant' in a statistical sense, the results can still be wrong or misleading. The best example of this problem is the matter of abortions and breast cancer. This was considered in Chapter 7, on reproductive risk factors, where it was shown that the most careful review of all the evidence gave 'significant' results indicating that induced abortions were a risk factor for breast cancer.[7] It was only as a consequence of a later study from Denmark that it was shown there was a 'systematic' error in the review.[8] 'Systematic' implies a recurring error due to the nature, system or environment in which most of the studies are conducted. In this case the consistent undercounting of the number of abortions led to the same error in most studies. The key exception was the Danish study, which was able to overcome the undercounting problem.

Care must also be taken when the results of a **single study** are considered in isolation. This is the opposite problem to the systematic error difficulty. As research workers seek financial support and recognition as well as enthusiasm for their projects, they often leap into the trap set by journalists by suggesting they have a 'breakthrough' cure for cancer or some other dreaded disease. Few of these claims, based on a single study, pass the test of time. Single studies may well offer accurate results, but may apply only to the study population and cannot be generalised to the whole world.

---

confidence interval a range of values within which results will lie with a specified probability
single study a study whose results have not been reproduced by other research workers

A good example is tobacco smoking. Single studies have strongly suggested that tobacco smoking increases the risk of coronary heart disease. However, nearly all these studies have been conducted on Western populations who for generations have consumed high levels of animal-based fats and for whom it is highly likely that tobacco does indeed increase coronary heart disease. But for populations like Japan, who do not consume high levels of animal fats, tobacco does not appear to carry such risks.

In the context of breast cancer we have already considered the possible influence of breastfeeding on risk. US-based studies have led to the conclusion that breastfeeding has no influence on risk of breast cancer. However, this only applies in the US context as studies in China show that breast cancer risk is probably reduced by breastfeeding. The unrecognised factor has been the prolonged nature of breastfeeding in China compared with the US.

Given these and other difficulties such as small sample sizes, inappropriate control groups, and the need to use indirect evidence in humans, some may question the validity of any results of research and will certainly challenge any dogmatic conclusions.

For these reasons, in recent years methods have been developed for considering the validity or otherwise of scientific evidence. These methods have become known as 'evidence-based medicine'. The essential feature of evidence-based medicine is that it is an organised systematic approach which considers the body of evidence as a whole in contrast to relying on the results of single studies in isolation. In addition, the evidence is rated according to the quality of the studies and the reliability of the methods used.

For example, a prospective study where the researchers are not permitted to know the identity of randomly selected patients who have been given a specific treatment is rated more highly than a study based on a series of observations on patients who were selected by the researcher. Such approaches are particularly useful when assessing the impact of an intervention such as lumpectomy instead of radical mastectomy for early breast cancer. In this case, the formal review of the evidence has shown that lumpectomy is as effective as radical mastectomy.

With respect to research aimed at finding the *cause* of a disease as distinct from a *treatment* for that disease, more complex approaches to assessing the strength of the evidence are required. The pioneer in this field is a British doctor, A. Bradford Hill, who developed a lifelong interest in the application of statistics to medical problems. Bradford Hill's approach is based on common sense. He raises a series of questions that challenge the evidence. Conclusions are based on a consideration of the questions and their answers as a whole.

Here are Bradford Hill's classic questions.

1 What is the strength and consistency of any associations?
2 Is there a relationship with age?
3 Are there any experimental results?
4 Are any associations or causal factors biologically plausible?
5 Is there a biological gradient?
6 Is there evidence for a specific cause?
7 Is the evidence coherent?
8 Is there any other way of explaining the facts?

Although the evidence relating to breast cancer has already been considered, it is helpful to reconsider this evidence as a whole using the Bradford Hill approach.

What is the strength and consistency of associations?

The strong correlation between per capita consumption of high-fat/high-calorie diets in specific countries and high rates of breast cancer has been constant since it was first observed more than 30 years ago.[9] Those countries with historically low rates of breast cancer, such as Japan, or intermediate rates, such as Italy, have experienced rises in breast cancer rates associated with increased consumption of fats/calories, whereas those countries that have long had high-fat/high-calorie diets have continued to experience high, but stable, rates of death due to breast cancer.[10,11] This can be regarded as Bradford Hill's 'biological gradient'—that is, the higher the national consumption of fats and energy the higher the incidence of breast cancer.

For more than 50 years it has been a consistent experience that the incidence and mortality rates for most cancers in migrants change from the rates of the originating country towards those of the host country.[12] When we look at breast cancer among migrants who have moved from countries with low risk of breast cancer to high-risk countries (which correlates with a move from countries with low consumption of fat/calories to high-consumption countries) the rates alter according to the overall differences between the originating and the host country, the period of residence in the host country, and whether born in the host country.

Is there any relationship with age?

The accumulating evidence that dietary experiences during pregnancy determine the hormonal environment of the foetus, and hence growth rates of the foetus, is compelling.[13] This evidence includes observations on humans (indirect evidence) and experimental evidence from animals (direct evidence).[14] At the present time there is no other explanation for the enormous differences in breast cancer risk between national populations.

Experiments with rodents offer compelling evidence that high-fat/high-calorie diets consumed by young (but not adult) animals are associated with a high risk of mammary tumours.[15–19] Therefore, there is an obvious incentive to seek parallels in human populations. A starting point is to observe the experiences of humans who migrate at young ages from low-risk countries to countries at high risk of breast cancer.[20,21]

Shimizu and colleagues have observed that Japanese who migrate at an early age develop higher rates of breast cancer than those who migrate at a late age, but that breast cancer rates for both these migrant groups is lower than for US-born Japanese.[20]

In the first study to evaluate directly the hypothesis that an early age at migration to the West exposes Asian women to Western lifestyles at a crucial age, Ziegler and colleagues found the risk of breast cancer declined steadily among women migrating at later ages.[21] It has also been shown that when Italian females from the south of Italy, who probably consumed low-fat/low-calorie diets, migrated to the north where higher-fat/higher-calorie diets were available, their risk of breast cancer increased. The younger the age of migration the greater the increase in risk.[22]

There is also a relationship between diet and age at menarche. Numerous factors acting in combination determine the age at menarche. These factors include genetic influences, exercise, health status and, above all, diet.[23-25]

The steady lowering of the age at menarche over the past 50 years and the associated rapid increase in height and weight of children and adults in many countries is probably due to changes in diet. Hill and colleagues showed that Caucasian girls from New York were 10–20% taller and heavier than Bantu girls from rural South Africa and their age at menarche was more than two years earlier.[26] Similar findings have come from Papua New Guinea.[27] The age at menarche in Japan has fallen from 16.4 to 14.4 years and in the US from 14.1 to 13.1 years between the years 1880 and 1944. These falls in age at menarche are correlated with increases in weight.[28] In Western countries menarche occurs earlier in overweight adolescents.[29]

In addition, diet appears to determine the age of achievement of maximum height, which in turn is associated with risk of breast cancer.[30] The earlier the age of reaching maximum height the greater the risk.

The association between age, exposure to radiation and breast cancer risk also provides strong evidence that young females are at increased susceptibility to influences that increase the risk of breast cancer compared with adult females.[31,32]

Are there any experimental results?

There are studies in laboratory mice and rats which clearly show that high-fat diets consumed during pregnancy by experimental rats and mice are associated with increased rates of mammary tumours in female offspring.

There is also compelling evidence that high-fat/high-calorie diets consumed by young, but not adult, experimental animals are associated with a high risk of mammary tumours.

Biological plausibility?

Breast cancer is clearly hormone-dependent. Bilateral **oophorectomy** before the age of 40 years in women is associated with a lifetime reduction in risk of about 50% compared with having a natural menopause.[33] Experimental animal studies in dogs have shown that oophorectomy before the first oestrus cycle almost totally removes the risk of breast cancer compared with dogs with intact ovaries.[34]

In turn, nutritional status has a direct effect on reproductive physiology in general, and on sex hormone production in particular. Women with anorexia nervosa cease to menstruate; high-fat/high-calorie diets are associated with early onset of menarche and late onset of menopause; such diets consumed in the peripubertal period increase the levels of sex hormones compared with young females on low-fat/low-calorie diets.

There is no doubt about the biological feasibility of intergenerational carcinogenic influences. The most dramatic instance

---

oophorectomy removal of the ovaries

of such influence is vaginal cancer in daughters of mothers who had taken artificial oestrogens.[35] Examples of more subtle influences are the increased risks of childhood leukaemia, Wilm's tumours, neuroblastomas, astrocytomas and testicular cancers in those who were large babies.[36,37]

Is there a biological gradient?

The ecological (population) evidence in humans and the experimental evidence in animals provide good support for the presence of a biological gradient with respect to energy consumption and breast cancer. In humans, countries with the highest per capita consumption of fats and calories have the highest risk of breast cancer. As per capita consumption of fats and calories rises in specific countries over a period of time, so does the risk of breast cancer. Similarly with experimental animals: as consumption of energy rises or falls so does the incidence of mammary tumours. There does, however, appear to be a possible threshold effect which has been observed in experimental animals.[38] *Threshold effect* means that there is an effect above or below a specific level of nutrition and that continued decreases or increases have no, or little, additional influence. There is no evidence available for such a threshold effect in humans, except the broad trends of national food consumption which are compatible with this theory. These broad trends suggest that if national consumption of daily calories is above 2800 per day, then the risk of breast cancer rises rapidly.

Of course, the association is more complicated than a simple dose response and appears to depend on a range of additional factors, including age, fertility, energy expenditure (exercise) and genetic susceptibility plus the composition of nutrients.

Is there evidence of a specific cause?

One of the major difficulties with the search for the causes of breast cancer has been the lack of a specific carcinogen—as, for example, tobacco in the case of lung cancer. However, there are several obvious specifics: breast cancer is overwhelmingly a gender-related cancer, there is a specificity in the magnitude of the association between breast cancer rates in populations who consume low-energy as compared with high-energy diets; and specific familial susceptibility to breast cancer is well established. In addition, there is a specific relationship beween alcohol consumption and breast cancer risk.

Is the evidence coherent?

The evidence that diet during pregnancy influences breast cancer risk in female offspring, and that high-fat/high-calorie diets, perhaps associated with little exercise, lead to early age at menarche, which in turn leads to increased risk of breast cancer, and that increased weight in the postmenopausal period increases risk offers a coherent theory or explanation for the underlying causes of breast cancer. There is evidence that there are additional risk factors—genetics, age at first full-term pregnancy and alcohol consumption.

Is there any other way of explaining the facts?

There is no evidence that viruses or other infectious agents are associated with breast cancer in humans despite the well known virus associated with mammary tumours in mice. There are no known chemicals, pesticides, metals or other substances associated with breast cancer. While there may be an association of exposure to electromagnetic fields and breast cancer, the evidence is equivocal and does not explain the global epidemiology of breast cancer. Plant oestrogens, which are found in soy beans, have been suggested as a contributing factor in the low rate of breast cancer in Asian populations, but this does not fit with other epidemiological observations.[39] Vitamin D has been suggested as an anti-carcinogenic compound but, again, this does not fit other evidence.[40] There is a modest protective effect of four antioxidant nutrients—vitamin A, vitamin C, vitamin E and possibly selenium—in low-risk countries but this has not been shown in high-risk countries.[40-42]

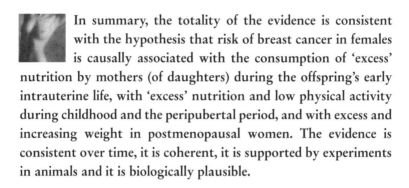 **In summary, the totality of the evidence is consistent with the hypothesis that risk of breast cancer in females is causally associated with the consumption of 'excess' nutrition by mothers (of daughters) during the offspring's early intrauterine life, with 'excess' nutrition and low physical activity during childhood and the peripubertal period, and with excess and increasing weight in postmenopausal women. The evidence is consistent over time, it is coherent, it is supported by experiments in animals and it is biologically plausible.**

Conclusions in detail

Maternal nutrition and breast cancer in offspring

The evidence to support the hypothesis that maternal nutritional experiences are an important influence on breast cancer risk in offspring is *limited* but compelling.

Childhood and adolescence

There is *sufficient* evidence to establish that early age at menarche is associated with subsequent increased risk of breast cancer by 5–10% for each year of reduction of the age at menarche. Early-age menarche is also associated with early-age onset of regular menstrual cycles, which in turn is associated with subsequent increased risk of breast cancer.

There is an association between an early age of achievement of maximum height, which is also associated with early-age menarche, and subsequent increased risk of breast cancer.

There is *sufficient* evidence to support the conclusion that age at menarche is determined by achievement of a common weight in a given society, which in turn is determined primarily by nutritional experiences in combination with expenditure of energy.

There is *insufficient* evidence to enable the development of detailed dietary and exercise guidelines for children and adolescents.

There is *limited* evidence that consumption of breast milk may be associated with a small reduction in risk of breast cancer. This may be because of the high energy in baby formulas of the 1950s and 1960s. Prolonged breastfeeding (more than two years) may offer some reduction in risk of breast cancer. This is based on observations in Chinese women. Breastfeeding for 6–9 months does not appear to offer any protection against breast cancer.

Adult women

▦ *Pregnancy*

There is *sufficient* evidence to confirm the one-third protection of a full-term pregnancy before the age of 20, compared with the age of 30 years. It is probable that a full-term pregnancy allows complete differentiation of breast calls, thereby protecting against cancer.

Short-term pregnancy followed by termination in the first trimester does not appear to influence risk of breast cancer. This firm conclusion is based on studies of women in Denmark where there is compulsory reporting of abortions. These findings differ from previous studies in countries where such reporting is voluntary. These findings also offer confirmation of the probable protective effect of complete differentiation of breast cells, which occurs during the third trimester of pregnancy.

■ *Nutrition, exercise and weight*
There is *sufficient* evidence to support the following conclusions: (1) excess weight during the premenopausal years is not associated with an increase in breast cancer risk; (2) fat consumption during adult life is not associated with increased risk; (3) excess rapid weight gain during the postmenopausal period is associated with increased risk ('rapid' means 4 kilos in 4 years).

There is *limited* evidence that monounsaturated fats, from sources such as olive oil, may offer some protection against breast cancer.

There is *limited* evidence to suggest that regular exercise may offer some protection against breast cancer.

■ *Alcohol*
There is *sufficient* evidence to establish a firm dose-related link between alcohol consumption and breast cancer risk.

possibilities for control and prevention

F ive very different approaches to the control of breast cancer have emerged during the past decade.

1 Early detection and treatment

By far the most common response to the challenge has been to conclude that the cause is unknown, and therefore prevention is not possible and priority must be given to early detection and treatment. To date this has been the most successful approach and has been responsible for the stabilisation and slight reduction in deaths due to breast cancer that have occurred in the US, UK, Canada, Australia and many other countries since 1989. However, despite these gains, the problem of breast cancer is huge and remains the most important malignancy in Western women.

2 Tamoxifen and other 'anti-oestrogens'

The second approach has been to develop pharmaceuticals such as the anti-oestrogen, tamoxifen, which alter hormone metabolism and reduce breast cancer risk.[1,2] These pharmaceuticals work by blocking the effect of natural oestrogens. During 1998 considerable publicity was given to the cessation of one US-based trial of tamoxifen; the results were so positive the researchers were concerned that it was unfair to restrict the pharmaceutical to the 'intervention' group of women and deny the benefits to the comparative group of women in the trial. A review of all 55 trials (studies) where tamoxifen has been given to women with early breast cancer was published in May 1998.[2] The results confirm the value of tamoxifen in improving the survival of women with early breast cancer.

However, the US study also identified a major problem. There was an increase among older women in the trials of three uncommon but serious disorders—endometrial cancer (cancer of the lining of the womb), pulmonary embolism (a large blood clot in the blood vessels supplying the lungs: a usually fatal complication) and deep vein thrombosis (a possibly fatal blockage of the main veins). Such serious side effects virtually eliminate the use of tamoxifen as a means of preventing breast cancer in normal women, but its use can be readily justified in women who already have cancer in one breast and need to prevent its occurrence in the other breast, and in other groups of women at high risk of breast cancer (e.g. women with a strong family history of the disease).

Fortunately, other potentially safer pharmaceuticals are being developed. The most developed of these is raloxifene. While the principle behind raloxifene is similar to tamoxifen, the focus for its use is on the prevention of osteoporosis, with protection from breast and endometrial cancer as a beneficial side effect. Raloxifene has been approved by the US authorities for the prevention of osteoporosis, and studies are under way to determine whether the early indications for such beneficial additional effects are confirmed.

3 Artificial pregnancies

The use of placental hormones in **nulliparous** women as a means of mimicking a full-term pregnancy and thereby reducing breast cancer

---

a **nulliparous** woman has never borne a child

risk has been explored in experimental animals and human breast cells. Early results suggest this may be possible but, again, the issue of safety is paramount.

4 Vitamin A-like substances

The use of vitamin A-like pharmaceuticals (retinoids) as a means of preventing breast cancer is being explored and early laboratory results are promising.[3] However, these substances have been associated with foetal damage in animals and, again, safety is a major issue.

5 Public health approaches

The public health approach has been the promotion of low-fat diets in adult women. Low-fat diet intervention trials were commenced in the early 1990s when current information suggested there was a relationship between consumption of fat and breast cancer.[4] It is now known that, for adults, there is almost certainly no direct link between total fat consumption and breast cancer and therefore such interventions are likely to have little impact. For children there is insufficient information to allow a definite answer. Total fat refers to all types of fat, including animal- and vegetable-sourced fats.

Several sound lessons, however, have been learned from these low-fat trials.[5]

The most important lesson has been the realisation that women regard the risk of breast cancer as much more important to them than other diseases such as coronary heart disease. Remember my wife Margaret's comment, 'I would much rather have a heart attack than get breast cancer.' The low-fat trials have shown that, where women perceive a risk of breast cancer, there is a fourfold greater reduction in their fat intake compared with other trials where the perceived risk was cardiovascular disease or heart attack. In other words, the fear of breast cancer has a much greater influence on women's health-related behaviour change than fear of heart disease.

It is probable that the use of hormone manipulation and vitamin-like substances to prevent breast cancer in whole populations contains far too many known and unknown risks to justify. These methods may, of course, have a role in selected women at high risk of breast cancer. Such women include those with a genetic tendency towards breast cancer, and those who have had breast cancer in one breast and are thus at increased risk of cancer in the other breast, and also spread of the cancer.

Therefore, approaches to the control and prevention of breast cancer which involve change in health-related behaviour should be a priority. Such approaches have the enormous advantages of safety, low cost, potential effectiveness and compatibility with other disease-prevention priorities such as cardiovascular disease and diabetes.

Some will argue with validity that there is insufficient evidence to justify the adoption of diets during pregnancy which are high in complex carbohydrates, fruit and vegetables and low in animal fats, as a means of avoiding very large babies who may be at subsequent increased risk of breast cancer. However, the evidence is equally lacking to justify the still common advice during pregnancy to 'eat for two' and 'milk and cheese are good for the baby's bones'. It is relevant to observe that Japanese mothers, who have the world's lowest infant mortality rates and the longest life span, consume low-fat, high-carbohydrate diets during pregnancy, and rarely consume dairy products.

The consumption of dairy products such as high-fat milk, cheese and icecream during pregnancy has become such a tradition, backed by earnest medical sages, that to suggest alternative diets may cause outrage and condemnation. However, the origins of the 'dairy food during pregnancy' tradition have been forgotten. It originated during the early part of the twentieth century when diseases associated with nutritional deficiencies were common. These included rickets which was associated with vitamin D deficiency, leading to malformation of the pelvis and other disorders of the bones. Dairy products were a good source of vitamin D and hence were encouraged. (Cod liver oil, herrings, sardines and tuna are rich sources of vitamin D.) The current problem is one of excess consumption of food, including dairy products, during pregnancy and, for that matter, during childhood.

Principles for primary prevention of breast cancer

It is not suggested that it is practical for Western women to attain the very low levels of breast cancer experienced in rural Asia. To do so would require a revolution in eating habits and reproductive behaviour over two or three generations. However, it is possible to modify the current risks by the adoption of a simple healthy lifestyle.

Based on current knowledge about breast cancer outlined in this book, a summary of suggested safe primary prevention approaches to breast cancer are:

1 the encouragement of breastfeeding, and of sound nutrition and regular exercise throughout life, but with particular emphasis on young age groups and pregnant women;
2 the avoidance of excess weight gain throughout adult life;
3 the consumption of alcohol in moderation;
4 encouragement of first full-term pregnancy before the approximate age of 28 years (but preferably at an even younger age).

There is insufficient evidence to offer details of what constitutes sound nutrition and regular exercise in the context of the prevention of breast cancer. However, women need specific advice on the adoption of a healthy lifestyle aimed at the prevention of breast cancer as well as a range of other relevant diseases such as coronary heart disease, stroke and diabetes. The suggestions that follow are as detailed as current knowledge allows.

Pregnancy

The advice often given to pregnant women to eat up on dairy products such as milk and cheese, as well as other high-energy foods such as animal-sourced fats and meats, is probably wrong. Such advice was based on traditional practices originating in days of absolute food shortages but remains in many national dietary guidelines.

The most practical advice for pregnant women is to eat plenty of cereals, fruit and vegetables and use meat, fish and poultry as garnishes rather than meals. While the evidence is incomplete, it is reasonable to increase the use of olive oil (high in monounsaturated fats) in place of cooking oils and fats sourced from dairy products, meats and plants that are high in saturated and polyunsaturated fats. In addition, regular exercise is a basic need to balance energy requirements.

If such a diet is readily available, there should be no need for vitamin supplements. However, if nausea or vomiting is a problem or if dietary patterns are not sound, then vitamin supplements, particularly folic acid (for the prevention of spinal deformities), can be important.

If you have a boy, you may think that all this healthy eating during the pregnancy was wasted and that avoiding those tempting chocolate gifts was not necessary. On the contrary, such efforts are probably even more worthwhile, because there is sound evidence that excess rich foods consumed during pregnancy may well be associated with subsequent increased risk of prostate cancer. This may seem even more fanciful than the possible prenatal origins of breast cancer, as prostate cancer tends to occur in old men. However, the biology is much the same as for breast cancer and the available evidence is very similar—namely, that big babies are at greater risk of prostate cancer than smaller babies!

Childhood

The same diet as for pregnant women is advised—namely, plenty of cereals, fruit and vegetables and avoidance of high-fat, high-energy foods such as potato chips, hamburgers, icecream and heavily sugared soft drinks. There is sound evidence that consumption of meat, rather than vegetables, nuts and cereals, will reduce the age at menarche by about 12 months and thereby modestly increase the subsequent risk of breast cancer.[6] Therefore, the encouragement of a low-fat diet (i.e. low in dairy products, meats and fatty fast foods) during childhood is advised.

For children and adolescents, regular exercise is an essential and simple way of balancing energy requirements and deferring menarche.

There is anecdotal evidence (evidence based on experience and not statistically valid) that if children and young people choose to reduce their consumption of energy and animal protein, and to exercise regularly, their age at menarche is readily deferred and excess weight does not become a problem. This is, of course, easy to preach and difficult to put into practice in an age of cheap icecream and hamburgers.

Adults

The message is the same as for pregnant women and children: plenty of cereals, fruit and vegetables and fewer fatty and heavily sugared foods.

Alcohol

There is no problem with regular but modest consumption of wine or beer. By 'modest' is meant no more than two drinks per day.

Age at first full-term pregnancy

First full-term pregnancy should be before the approximate age of 28 years, but preferably at a younger age.

This is realistic, despite the strong trend towards deferral of first child. For many women, careers have become essential to their fulfilment but, however difficult, it is possible to have babies plus a career. Just have the babies early! In the modern era of obstetrics, having a baby at any age is very safe but there are real disadvantages in having a late first baby, including of course an increase in risk of breast cancer. The additional disadvantages include a small risk of a baby with Down syndrome and the social problems of being comparatively old when the baby becomes a teenager.

Breastfeeding

Babies should be breastfed, but for how long? Certainly, there is no need to breastfeed for years, as in traditional societies, but longer than three months is highly desirable. Maybe 9–12 months is a reasonable compromise; after all, mother and baby have only this one opportunity for the rest of their lives. We do not want guilt to be part of mothering, but with the passing of years many women express remorse at having given up breastfeeding too early, or for not being able to establish it in the first place.

The reasons for not breastfeeding are obviously varied, and often multiple. Some women find breastfeeding exceedingly difficult—cracked nipples and a hungry baby can be a painful combination. Others find that financial restraints force them back into the workforce.

However, it is a sad reality that the decision to give up breastfeeding very early, or not to breastfeed at all, can affect the health and well-being of both mother and child.

What is a reasonable lifelong dietary pattern?

The aim is to achieve a lifelong eating pattern and not to 'diet'. All diets must end and most will be unsuccessful in the long term.

The simple answer is to copy the food traditions of southern Europeans and North, South and Eastern Asians. Their eating patterns are characterised by high consumption of cereals, either rice or wheat, and plenty of vegetables, with fish, chicken, meat and dairy products as garnishes rather than meals. Add as much fruit as desired. Olive oil is a staple cooking oil in southern European countries and a major source of monounsaturated fats. Although there is insufficient evidence on which to base dogmatic recommendations, because olive oil and monounsaturated fats are firmly associated with a reduction in risk of coronary heart disease, it is a safe and reasonable suggestion for the possible reduction in breast cancer risk.

Once such a pattern of food consumption is established, quantities do not matter, within reason, and there is no need for 'prescription dieting', providing we participate in regular daily exercise. An added bonus is that in most countries the adoption of such food consumption patterns is less costly than eating meat, biscuits and heavily sugared soft drinks.

There is no problem with eating festival foods during festivals— Christmas, birthdays, new year, wedding anniversaries and the like—but there is a problem with having festival foods every day. The transition from healthy traditional diets to consumption on a daily basis of festival foods, characterised by a high content of meat, animal fats and sugars, is typical of migrants and populations in countries that are experiencing rapid economic development. There is very little that can be done about this evolution except to provide information.

Osteoporosis and anorexia nervosa

We should not let issues such as osteoporosis and anorexia nervosa divert our attention from sensible food consumption. Of course, these conditions are of concern, but not to the extent of diseases such as breast cancer, coronary heart disease and diabetes which are experienced so commonly in Western countries.

Sensible exercise

In modern societies the need for heavy physical work has all but disappeared and as a consequence deliberate effort has to be made to exercise on a regular basis. But how much exercise? Marathon and triathlon competitors are unsuitable role models as their exertions are excessive from the perspective of a busy teenager or professional woman. On the other hand, confining activity to movements between the refrigerator and the television is equally unsuitable.

Half an hour *each day* spent walking, jogging or working out in the pool or gym, or in an aerobics group—or the equivalent expenditure of energy during work activities—is reasonable for women of all ages. This half-hour of exercise need not be completed in one session but can be spread throughout the day. Such physical activities can be social and very pleasant; they allow you to eat a bit more and yet keep a sound energy balance.

Oral contraceptives and postmenopausal hormone therapy

There is a slight increase in risk of breast cancer associated with current but not past use of oral contraceptives.

The current use of hormone replacement therapy (HRT) probably increases the risk of breast cancer in middle class Western women by

30–40% after five years of use. To get this in perspective, this increase in risk means that for every 1000 women who began use of HRT at age 50 years, and used it for 5, 10 and 15 years respectively, an additional 2, 6 and 12 women get breast cancer. On the other hand, such use reduces the risk of coronary heart disease by about the same proportion and may reduce the risk of stroke. HRT certainly reduces the risk of osteoporosis.

The menopause is a vulnerable time for many women. They may feel their body is 'falling apart' and may also be concerned about their relationship with spouse or partner. They may experience a major loss of self-confidence. HRT can help overcome these problems.

No specific guide can be offered about HRT, but for many women it may be worth considering for about five years after menopause. Such use will give some relief from symptoms of the menopause, and female characteristics that are hormone-dependent will be retained for an additional period. The risks from breast cancer are quite small for such limited use.

The best advice is to see your own doctor and seek an individual assessment. A knowledge of the information outlined in this book will place you in a good position for an informed discussion with your doctor.

Older women

Most readers of this book will have passed the opportunity of modifying the risk of breast cancer, either because their mothers were advised to eat milk, cheese and meat 'for two' when they conceived and nurtured you through pregnancy, or because you joined your teenage friends enjoying milkshakes and icecream and had an early menarche. This is far from being your fault—we all followed the same patterns of behaviour, and cancer was seen as a terrible thing that happened to other people in old age.

You can do nothing about the past, but you can do a great deal about the future. There are a number of very practical actions that all women over the age of 20 years can take. The first is not to defer your first baby into your thirties. The second is to get plenty of regular, pleasant exercise. The third is to adopt a lifelong pattern of eating a healthy diet, high in cereals, with fish, poultry and meat mainly as garnishes, plenty of fruit and vegetables, and low in fat and sugar. The fourth is to enjoy alcoholic drinks in moderation. The fifth and equally important action is to have regular mammograms from the age of about 50 years.

Finally, you can help to prevent breast cancer in your daughters. Although research evidence about the influence of nutrition during pregnancy is nowhere near 'proven', it is likely that 'excess nutrition' during pregnancy by mothers and grandmothers does influence the risk of breast cancer in daughters, and it is prudent to adopt sensible and safe prevention measures. These measures are to avoid 'excess nutrition' as outlined above, and to take regular, but not excessive, exercise throughout pregnancy. The new baby should be breastfed for at least 9–12 months and should be nourished throughout childhood and adolescence by the same nutritional approaches. Children and particularly adolescents should participate in regular, but not excessive, pleasant exercise.

Not only are these steps all very simple, very safe, affordable and absolutely achievable by everybody, they will help you reduce breast cancer and the full range of 'lifestyle' diseases (diabetes, coronary heart disease, stroke, gall bladder stones, colon cancer) that plague modern societies.

what can I do now?

We shared the review of breast cancer outlined in this book with women of all ages. Their responses varied, but they offered similar comments about the key prevention issues. The immediate response of all readers is to consider: 'How will this affect me?' They then take a broader view and begin to think about action that may reduce the risk in their children. Finally, they express disappointment that there is no simple solution such as a pill or a vaccine. Some readers directed anger at the research community for not communicating with the general public and sharing the solid facts about breast cancer that have become available.

Not all readers were interested in the personalities of the epidemiologists and other researchers who have created the new knowledge—they simply wanted to know what is required to prevent breast cancer. There are two good reasons why this reaction is disappointing. The first, very practical reason is that, unless there is continued support from the community, taxpayers' funds will be directed elsewhere, maybe into weaponry or other destructive research priorities. The second reason is that recognition provides an incentive to research scientists. Their work is far from glamorous and the outcome of most research is negative. The public tends to learn only of the success stories. There is little excitement in spending 20 vital years discovering that fibre, coffee and vitamin E are not causes of breast cancer.

On the other hand, the response from many women was very positive. For example, some readers are already setting out to have babies earlier than they had planned, others are reconsidering hormone replacement therapy and there is general acceptance of the need to maintain a sensible diet and exercise pattern at all ages.

Diet during pregnancy is a difficult issue for most readers because of the conflicting messages. The new knowledge outlined in this book, which suggests that dietary moderation and regular exercise during pregnancy will lead to healthy offspring, is in conflict with experiences of unhealthy babies following the deprivation of food in pregnant women. These views are understandable but are based on extreme situations, such as famine associated with war and civil disruption, and not on the normal lives of most readers.

There is another problem. This is the widespread belief that dieting as a means of weight reduction and control does not work. This belief is soundly based, as it is known that more than half the women in Western populations have participated at some stage in unsuccessful weight reduction programs. The incentive for women to maintain a low body weight is based mainly on appearance rather than health. However, this situation is rapidly changing. As we mentioned earlier, new studies have clearly shown that women dieting in an effort to reduce risk of breast cancer achieved a fourfold greater reduction in fat consumption than when the incentive was to reduce the risk of a heart attack.

These are very interesting new findings, because they show that women are able and willing to adopt a healthy diet so as to reduce the risk of breast cancer, whereas they are not so keen to do so to avoid other health problems.

We must distinguish the practice of 'dieting' from the adoption of healthy eating. Crash diets and fad diets usually involve the removal of fluids from the diet, or confine food intake to measured quantities. Such dieting is often futile in the long term, and should not be confused with the consumption of a healthy diet—characterised by high quantities of complex carbohydrates such as rice or wheat-based cereals, plenty of fruit and vegetables, lean meat and fish as garnishes and low animal and other fats. Such a diet can be consumed in virtually any amount and, provided it is combined with exercise, there is little chance of becoming overweight.

How to eat more fruit and vegetables

___

- Try one new fruit or vegetable each week.
- Double the normal serving size for vegetables.
- Eat fruit on cereal or muesli—bananas, apples, grapes, berries, peaches, mandarins.
- Have all-vegetable-based meals such as vegetable stews.
- Eat fruit as a snack.
- Drink fruit juice instead of 'soft' drinks.
- Have baked fruit for dessert, such as apple, peach, pear, banana.
- Take raw fruit and vegetable platters to parties.
- Eat more international dishes such as Oriental stir fries, Indian vegetable curries, Greek moussaka.

___

Source: Steinmetz KA, Potter JD, Vegetables, fruit, and cancer prevention: a review, J Am Diet Asoc 1996; 96: 1027–39.

Expectations

The expectation that it will be easy to prevent breast cancer, because the basic risk factors are now known, is wrong. As the risk factors mainly involve behaviour such as nutrition, exercise and age at first birth, and prevention involves modifying such behaviour, any reduction in risk for whole populations will be difficult to achieve. Even a reduction in risk by individuals will not be easy.

___

Take Elizabeth, as an unfortunate example. She was always slim, she was physically active all her life, had her first child when she was 22 and had no family history of breast cancer, and yet she developed fatal breast cancer.

___

But we must not finish on such a sad note. Despite the formidable challenge of breast cancer, it is possible for all girls and all women to take specific actions that will, to some extent, reduce their risk and that of their offspring of developing breast cancer. These actions are free of cost, safe and can be commenced immediately.

What can I do now?

Given the fact that breast cancer is both serious and common, it is absolutely natural for most women to be anxious and concerned. Some argue that as breast cancer is rare in young women, they should not be concerned until they pass the age of 40 years. However, rare events still happen and in our view care should be taken at all ages.[1,2]

Action tends to relieve anxiety. If you are an adult, however, exercise, diet, and alcohol restriction (while worth the effort) can offer only modest levels of protection. Also, you may already be over the age when a pregnancy will offer protection. So, in addition to these basic prevention measures, early diagnosis and early treatment must be paramount.

Early diagnosis

Regular physical examination of the breasts by both yourself and a doctor or other health professional is a good start. It is best to do a simple breast self-examination just after your period finishes. At the end of menstruation there are fewer normal swellings and thickenings of the tissues of the breast than at any other time during the monthly cycle and, therefore, there is less chance of confusing normal with abnormal changes in the breast. If you no longer have periods, simply choose a day each month that is easy to remember such as the first Sunday in the month. It is also reasonable to have a breast examination by a doctor at yearly intervals as part of an annual check-up (use your birthday as a convenient reminder).

There are two signs to look for during breast self-examination:

1 any discharge of fluid from the nipple
2 any small lumps or thickenings of the breast tissue.

Self-examination is probably best done while you are having a bath or shower as water and soap make it easy to examine the whole breast gently with the fingers. However, breast self-examinations can be readily conducted while standing in front of a mirror or lying down in bed.

Use the flat of your fingers rather than the fingertips. Gently move your fingers in circles and feel each part of both breasts. It is best to put one hand behind your head while examining the breast with the other hand. This stretches the muscles behind the breast and makes it easier to examine. Check your nipples for any changes. There should be a small hollow behind the nipples. Then check right up into your armpits.

Do not expect to make a diagnosis yourself as you do not have the experience to do so. All you are aiming to do is to recognise the presence of a change in your breast, or a new small lump or thickening, and then to seek advice.

If you do identify a new lump or a change in an old lump or any thickening of the breast tissue, you will inevitably be worried. That is a completely normal reaction and you must not be concerned about going to the doctor with a problem that turns out to be nothing. Fortunately, 95% of such lumps and thickenings turn out to be normal and are not breast cancer. Don't feel embarrassed that the lump is normal, or that you have bothered the doctor for nothing—you have a responsibility to your family and friends to seek medical advice and doctors have a responsibility to check whether there is a problem.

Similarly, a liquid discharge from the nipple is likely to be due to a minor infection or hormonal change, but again you have a responsibility to check.

The outlook for women with breast cancer is better if the problem is diagnosed early, so it is crucial not to defer an examination by a doctor, or a mammogram. However, many highly intelligent and otherwise practical people put off going to the doctor. The most compelling reason is fear of the unknown. Both men and women fear the doctor will find something wrong, and perhaps unconsciously overcome the fear by taking no action. Other reasons include concern about the examinations and tests.

If you are such a person and you are worried, you are in very good company. The late Professor Derek Llewellyn Jones continually deferred seeking help for possible prostate cancer until it was too late. Professor Jones was a sophisticated gynaecologist who wrote the immensely popular book *Everywoman*, which included advice to women to seek early help if they were worried about breast cancer. His last published words were: 'If only I had sought early help, but I could not cope with the idea of a rear-end digital examination!' This was a sad farewell from a doctor who had performed thousands of such examinations on women.

Mammograms

A mammogram is an X-ray of the breast which can diagnose very small breast cancers, even if they are as small as a grain of rice. The dose of the X-ray is very small and is therefore reasonably safe.

During a mammogram, the breast is flattened between the two plates of the X-ray machine for several seconds. The X-ray picture is then reviewed by a specialist.

It is wise to have a mammogram every two years after the age of 40 years and once a year after the age of 50 years. Mammography has revolutionised the early diagnosis of breast cancer and you should take advantage of its value. About 90% of breast cancers can be diagnosed by this examination. However a mammogram does not guarantee freedom from breast cancer, either at the time of the examination or during the period between mammograms. Therefore breast self-examinations and medical check-ups are essential.

Why are 95% of breast lumps normal?

The most common reason for having lumps or thickenings in the breast is hormonal changes as part of the menstrual cycle. Unfortunately, it can be difficult to distinguish such changes from early cancer and this is the reason for being so careful to observe any abnormal changes.

Hormonal changes during the cycle can lead to swollen and tender breasts. Such discomfort, and even pain, is rarely a sign of cancerous change. It can be useful to keep a written record, even a simple diagram, of such breast symptoms over several months to determine whether they are part of the cycle.

Hormonal changes can also lead to the formation of soft lumps and thickening of the breast tissue. Again, the keeping of a written record or diagram can help in excluding anything abnormal.

Fibroadenomas

Many younger women have smooth firm lumps in the breast made up of fibrous and glandular tissue. These lumps may become more tender in the days before a period or during pregnancy. The reason for the development of such lumps is not known. They are not cancerous and rarely change into breast cancer.

Most younger women should not have fibroadenomas removed, unless the adenoma enlarges. Removal requires simple surgery.

Cysts

A cyst is a sac full of fluid in the breast. During the menstrual cycle, fluid is produced and then absorbed. Some women are more susceptible than others to developing such cysts. Breast cysts are more common in women aged 35–50 years than in younger women. They are also common in women taking hormone replacement therapy.

Simple cysts are not cancerous nor do they change into breast cancer.

Investigation and diagnosis

If breast self-examination or a clinical examination (an examination carried out by a doctor or other health professional) or a mammogram detects a lump or thickening in the breast which is causing some concern, it becomes necessary to investigate the situation. Such investigation is undertaken through a series of simple steps.

Step 1 Clinical breast examination

A clinical breast examination involves a thorough examination of the whole breast area, including the armpits and the front of the chest. With all the woman's upper clothing removed, the doctor looks at the breasts while she is seated or standing to see if any changes to the breast are present. Following this observation the doctor examines both breasts and nipples.

Always included in a clinical breast examination is the taking of a clinical history. This involves a series of questions concerning age, family history of breast and other cancers, menstrual and reproductive history (such as how many babies and at what age you had them), whether you have swelling and discomfort of the breasts during the menstrual cycle, alcohol consumption levels, and whether you are taking oral contraceptives or hormone replacement therapy.

Very often, the clinical history and examination will be part of a general medical check-up and therefore not solely concerned with breast cancer. In this case, the history, examination and any tests will be more comprehensive than if only breast cancer is being considered.

If you have detected a lump or change in your breasts the doctor will seek to determine if these changes are due to normal changes. The process follows a logical series of questions:

■ *Are the changes hormonal?*
This can be assessed by asking (a) when, during the menstrual cycle, did you note changes in the breast? (b) have your periods been regular during recent months? (c) have you started, stopped or changed hormone replacement therapy or oral contraceptives? (These alter hormone levels and can be the cause of changes in the breast.)

   If the doctor's assessment is that the changes in your breast are due to hormonal factors then no further tests or examinations are necessary at this time, although follow-up in several months time is advisable.

■ *Are any changes in the breast part of the normal breast structure?*
The shape and feel of normal breasts change over time and at different times. Sometimes, the doctor will be able to indicate that the breast changes are most likely normal tissues. Such normal tissues may feel a little different from the rest of the breast tissue or may even be an underlying rib.

   If the doctor's assessment is that any breast changes are normal then further tests and examinations are not required at this time. However, if you feel the lump or other changes again during the next 2–3 months, you should return for another clinical examination.

■ *Could it be a cancerous breast lump?*

A lump that is breast cancer usually has a different feel from a lump caused by a cyst or fibroadenoma, or by changes in breast tissue associated with the menstrual cycle. If such a lump feels hard, has an irregular shape or is attached to other parts of the breast or skin or muscle, then it is likely to be breast cancer. If there is any such suspicion you will need to have further tests to confirm or deny the diagnosis.

Step 2 Imaging tests

The next step is to have an imaging test. There are two types of imaging tests: mammography and ultrasound. Both tests may be needed.

■ *Mammogram*

In addition to the use of mammograms as a means of early diagnosis of breast cancer, they are also useful if breast cancer is suspected. More detailed mammograms can be very helpful by providing extra information about the lump prior to any surgery.

■ *Ultrasound*

An ultrasound test is the same in principle as a mammogram except that sound waves are used to form an image of the breast and any cancerous changes. Ultrasound tests are particularly useful for distinguishing between cancer and cysts.

The results of these imaging tests determine whether further tests are needed. However, it should be known that such imaging tests cannot give an absolute guarantee that there is no cancer present. On the other hand, imaging tests are helpful in avoiding much unnecessary surgery to remove lumps from the breast which in most cases are normal.

Step 3 Needle biopsy or core aspiration

If breast cancer cannot be reasonably excluded by the imaging tests, it may be necessary to proceed to a needle or core biopsy. The difference between a needle biopsy and a core biopsy is that only a few cells are removed by needle whereas a piece, or core, of tissue is removed in the core biopsy. These cells and tissues can then be examined by microscope and a diagnosis of cancer can be confirmed. On the other hand, these tests cannot exclude breast cancer and the next step may have to be taken.

Step 4 Open surgical biopsy

This test is the 'gold standard' for the diagnosis of breast cancer. The open biopsy can be used to confirm or deny the presence of cancer. As for all medical matters, open biopsy is not absolutely accurate or foolproof but its reliability is very high. Open biopsy obviously leaves a scar and there can be some minor discomfort, but it is a very safe procedure.

Investigations of changes to the nipple

The key changes to the nipple that are associated with breast cancer are discharge of fluid, inversion of the nipple, ulcers of the nipple and changes in colour.

▪ *Fluid* that contains blood, fluid that comes from a single duct in one nipple, fluid that comes out without squeezing the breast, and fluid that is a new discharge in a postmenopausal woman may all indicate the possibility of breast cancer. If any of these changes occurs it is important to have the series of tests outlined above.

■ *Nipple inversion.* Inversion means that the nipple grows inwards instead of outwards. If such inversion is a new change, the investigations above are needed.

What to do if breast cancer is diagnosed

If you are diagnosed as having breast cancer you obviously face a serious problem, but it is not the end of the world. Many cancers of the breast are very treatable and the outlook can be quite good, particularly if the diagnosis is made at an early stage. In addition, and most importantly, modern treatment usually involves **lumpectomy** where the tumour is removed and the breast is left largely intact.

If it is confirmed that you have breast cancer, anticipate going through the processes of grief. These stages of grief are well known and completely normal. They begin with denial of the problem which is soon replaced with feelings of anger—the 'why me?' reaction. After a period of several weeks, or even some months, acceptance follows and this can lead to positive planning for the future. No one finds these processes easy—they are highly emotional and difficult to handle.

Throughout the grieving process, life is made easier if you can share the problem with others, particularly those who have special meaning for you such as your husband or partner, and other members of your family and friends, including your children. You will probably find that family, friends and work colleagues will have difficulty handling the situation; they will not know whether you wish to keep the matter private or to have a chat about things. It may help to indicate to them what your wishes are—either discreetly to discuss the problem or to keep it to yourself.

Many people will offer help when you do not really need any. A good way to handle this is to say something like: 'I'm anxious about

---

lumpectomy removes the tumour, leaving the breast largely intact

my problem but with time I shall cope. There is no need for help but I'm having some difficulty balancing work and the new medical commitments so if you could make a cake or a simple meal that I can share, it would be very nice.' Not only is such an approach diplomatic, but it gives the kindly person an idea of how to help in a small way, and will give both of you great satisfaction. Such practical help can be valuable during a difficult time—it is hard enough coping with newly diagnosed breast cancer without having to cook the dinner!

It is beyond the scope of this book to explore in detail the treatment methods available for breast cancer. However, it is important for you to know that treatment methods are continually improving and that the outlook for people with breast cancer, while serious, has never been better. In addition, the international research effort into new and more effective ways of treating breast cancer has reached a very promising stage.

glossary

aggressiveness how quickly a cancer spreads.

anatomy the gross structure of the body and parts of the body.

anecdotal evidence evidence based on personal experience. Such evidence may not be reliable.

anovular when no ovulation occurs.

anti-angiogenesis action against the growth of new blood vessels. This is a new term used in the context of developing substances that retard the growth of blood vessels which supply nutrients to cancers.

antioxidants substances that inhibit oxidation. Oxidation is a chemical process involving oxygen and leading to the breakdown of substances. Antioxidants may be associated with the protection of genetic material in cells and ensure safe, regulated cell multiplication. Vitamin E is an example of an antioxidant, but has not been shown to influence breast cancer risk.

axilla (pl. axillae) the armpit, the most common place for the initial spread of breast cancer.

biopsy removal of a piece of tissue from the body for examination, usually under a microscope.

breast cancer the breast is a modified gland of the skin containing the cells that secrete milk for the nourishment of the young. Breast cancer is a malignant change in various parts of the breast. The most common (about 90% of breast cancers) is malignant change of the linings of the small milk ducts; much less common is malignant change of the large milk ducts (about 5%) and the milk-producing cells (about 5%).

calorie a unit of heat or energy. Main sources of calories are fats and carbohydrates. Attempts are being made to replace the term with *kilojoule*. One calorie is equivalent to about 4 kilojoules.

cancer cells that become invasive. That is, their growth becomes uncontrolled and they invade surrounding tissues, blood and lymphatic systems. When specialised cells become cancerous or malignant they change to an appearance like the cells seen in an embryo. It is these changes in the appearance of cells that allows the diagnosis of cancer to be made.

The terms *malignancy* and *neoplasm* are interchangeable with cancer.

carbohydrates chemicals made of carbon, hydrogen and oxygen in a form that can be converted to energy and water. Cereals and vegetables have a high carbohydrate content. They can be a major source of energy for the body.

carcinogen a carcinogen triggers cancerous changes in a cell.

cardiovascular disease diseases of the heart and blood vessels. Usually, the term is used when discussing the progressive thickening of the blood vessels that is commonly associated with fatty diets.

case-control study a research method which compares the characteristics of people with a disease such as breast cancer (cases) with similar aged people who do not have breast cancer (controls). While such methods are useful, the results can be biased because of difficulty in selecting strictly comparable groups for study.

causal helping to cause a disease.

cell the most fundamental unit of the body. It consists of a round nucleus containing genetic material, surrounded by cytoplasm which contains nutrients to support the nucleus. The cell is enclosed in a membrane. Multiple collections of cells make up tissues such as muscle.

cell nucleus a round body in the centre of a cell containing genetic material. It is this genetic material that becomes malignant or cancerous.

cervical cancer cancer of the neck of the womb.

chemotherapy treatment with chemicals or pharmaceuticals that attack cancer cells in preference to normal cells. Chemotherapy is often associated with severe side effects such as nausea, loss of hair and bleeding of the gums.

chromosomes the genetic material in all cells of the body.

circumstantial evidence such evidence implies an association between a factor and the disease being studied, but the factor may not be causal.

confidence interval (CI) a range of values within which results will lie with a specified probability. The usual probability is that there is a 95% likelihood that the values are accurate.

cyst a sac full of fluid.

dizygotic twins non-identical twins.

endometrial cancer cancer of the lining of the womb.

epidemiologist a scientist who uses epidemiologic techniques.

epidemiology the use of statistical techniques to study patterns of disease and injury in populations and communities.

familial affecting several members of the same family A familial disease or condition may or may not be hereditary.

fats chemicals that can form the familiar fatty substance in the body. Fats exist in many forms and have different influences according to their chemical structure. *Monounsaturated fats*, found in olive oil, appear to reduce risk of coronary heart disease and maybe breast cancer. *Polyunsaturated fats*, as found in vegetable margarines, may be associated with increased risk of breast cancer. *Saturated fats*, as found in dairy products and fatty meats, do not appear to influence breast cancer but increase risk of coronary heart disease.

foetus the product of conception. At about 22–24 weeks' gestation the foetus becomes viable (able to live outside the womb) and the term *unborn infant* or *baby* is commonly used.

genetic material the biological unit of heredity. It is self-reproducing and hence fundamental to growth in general and cancerous growth in particular.

genetics the study of heredity.

gestation time since conception of the foetus.

growth hormone a chemical substance carried in the blood that influences the growth of most tissues of the body.

histopathology examination of tissues under a microscope. The 'gold standard' for the diagnosis of breast cancer.

hormone replacement therapy the replacement of natural hormones by artificial hormones, usually after the menopause.

hormones there are many different hormones. They are chemicals secreted by glands such as the thyroid (in the neck), the pituitary (in the base of the brain), the adrenals (on top of the kidneys) and of course the ovaries (in the lower pelvis). These chemicals influence growth, reproduction, sex, heartbeat and body temperature.

hypothesis idea based on limited evidence, awaiting proof.

incidence the extent of occurrence of a disease in a given population.

intervention the giving of treatment.

invasive describes a cancer that has spread into local (nearby) tissues.

late stage promotion influences on the later stages of the development of cancer.

lumpectomy removal of a breast cancer, leaving the breast intact.

lymphatic system a system of very small ducts that carries lymph. *Lymph* is a yellowish fluid containing small cells known as *lymphocytes,* which are part of the defensive system of the body against infection. The lymphatic system can be invaded by cancer cells. Breast cancer often spreads to the axilla via the lymphatic system. The lymphatic system contains lymph nodes—small nodules 1–25 mm in diameter which can be readily found in the armpits or groin. Their purpose is to manufacture and store lymphocytes which are part of the body's defensive mechanism.

malignant describes a cancer which has the potential for uncontrollable growth and spread.

mammary tumour a tumour in the breast.

mammography X-ray examination of the breasts for cancer.

mastectomy complete removal of the breast.

melanoma cancer of the pigment-forming cells of the skin. Usually caused by excessive exposure to the sun by fair people.

menarche the onset of menstruation.

menopause the cessation of menstrual cycles.

meta-analysis review of a number of studies, usually by combining the original data.

metastasis spread of cancer, usually via the blood vessels or lymphatic system.

micronutrients nutrients present in food in tiny but often essential amounts.

microscope a magnifying instrument used for examining tissues to determine whether they have malignant characteristics.

nulliparous describes a woman who has never borne a child.

oestrogen one of the most influential female hormones. Oestrogens influence the deposition of fat on the body to give the familiar female form, they are involved in the menstrual cycle and are necessary for the development of breast cancer—no oestrogens, no breast cancer.

oncologist a medical practitioner who specialises in the treatment of cancer.

oophorectomy removal of the ovaries.

osteoporosis fragile bones due to loss of calcium.

outcome the results of a research study or treatment.

ovaries the female glands situated in the lower pelvis, which produce ova (eggs) and a range of female hormones including oestrogen.

parenchyma the specific cells of the breast contained in a connective tissue framework. Seen as shadows in X-rays.

parity number of pregnancies.

pathologist a medical practitioner who specialises in laboratory work in general and in the diagnosis of cancer by use of microscopes.

perimenarcheal around the time of menarche.

peripubertal around the time of puberty.

phytoestrogens oestrogens sourced from plants.

pilot intervention usually an experimental action, a trial of a new treatment.

placebo a medicine that has no effect.

population small or large group of people, selected to take part in a study.

postmenopausal after the cessation of menstrual cycles.

postulate put forward an idea.

premenopausal before the onset of menopause.

prenatal before birth.

primary prevention preventing the occurrence of disease processes. For example: primary prevention of high blood pressure involves preventing the problem from ever happening; secondary prevention of high blood pressure concerns its treatment so as to avoid complications such as stroke.

prospective study a research method that studies the characteristics of people before they develop a disease such as breast cancer. Such studies reduce the bias inherent in selecting groups for comparison, as in case-control studies.

proteins complex chemicals made up of sequences of amino acids. Alter the sequence and the function of the proteins also alters. Hormones are largely made of proteins. Proteins are involved in the transport of oxygen, muscle contraction, and a range of body functions.

radiation high-energy electromagnetic rays, like a focused X-ray.

radiation therapy treatment with radiation. The principle is the same as for chemotherapy. The side effects can be similar.

significant used by scientists to have a specific statistical meaning. If the results from a research study are 'statistically significant', they are not due to chance or luck. Such significance is given added meaning by indicating that there is a 95% probability that the result is true and a 5% chance that the result is due to chance. *See also* **confidence interval**.

single study a research study that has not been confirmed by other similar studies.

socioeconomic status status measured or assessed according to a range of defined factors such as education, income, occupation and place of residence.

toxins substances that are harmful.

trauma damage to the body. It may be caused by a wide range of factors, such as a car accident, a punch, a fall or scratching an itchy nose.

ultrasound the use of sound waves to produce an image. This is a very safe technique commonly used in the diagnosis of cysts in the breast.

undifferentiated describes cancers comprising primitive or non-specialised cells. Such cancers are often fast growing and potentially lethal.

references

1 ELIZABETH SUTHERLAND

1 Fisher B, Bauer M, Margolese R, et al. Five-year results of a randomized clinical trial comparing total mastectomy and segmental mastectomy with or without radiation in the treatment of breast cancer. N Engl J Med 1985; 312: 665–73.

2 WHAT IS BREAST CANCER?

1 Hilakivi-Clarke L. Mechanisms by which high maternal fat intake during pregnancy increases breast cancer risk in female rodent offspring. Breast Cancer Research Treatment 1997; 46: 199–214.

2 De Waard F, Baanders-van Halewijn EA, Huizinga J. The bimodal age distribution of patients with mammary carcinoma. Cancer 1963; 17: 141–51.

3 Yong L-C, Brown CC, Schatzkin A, Schairer C. Prospective study of relative weight and risk of breast cancer: the breast cancer detection demonstration project follow up study, 1979 to 1987–1989. Am J Epidemiol 1996; 143: 985–95.

4 Hunter DJ, Willett WC. Diet, body size and breast cancer. Epidemiol Rev 1993; 15: 110–32.

5 Ursin G, Longnecker MP, Haile RW, Greenland S. A meta-analysis of body mass index and risk of premenopausal breast cancer. Epidemiology 1995; 6: 137–41.

6 Hall JM, Lee MK, Newman B, Morrow JE, Anderson LA, Huey B, King M-C. Linkage of early-onset familial breast cancer to chromosome 17q21. Science 1990; 250: 1686–9.

7 Colditz GA, Willett WC, Hunter DJ, et al. Family history, age and risk of breast cancer. JAMA 1993; 270: 338–43.

8 Colditz GA, Rosner BA, Speizer FE. Risk factors for breast cancer according to family history of breast cancer. J Natl Cancer Inst 1996; 88: 365–71.

9 Yuan JM, Yu MC, Ross RK, Gao YT, Henderson BE. Risk factors for breast cancer in Chinese women in Shanghai. Cancer Res 1988; 49: 1949–53.

10 Tao SC, Yu MC, Ross RK, Xiu KW. Risk factors for breast cancer in Chinese women in Beijing. Int J Cancer 1988; 42: 495–8.

11 Parkin DM, Whelan SL, Ferlay J, Raymond L, Young J. Cancer incidence in five continents. IARC 1997. Scientific Publication 143, Lyons.

12 MacMahon B, Cole P, Brown J. Etiology of human breast cancer. J Natl Cancer Inst 1973; 50: 21–42.

13 Boyd NF, Martin LJ, Noffel M, Lockwood GA, Tritchler DL. A meta-analysis

of studies of dietary fat and breast cancer risk. Br J Cancer 1993; 68: 627–36.

14 Howe GR, Hirohata T, Hislop TG, et al. Dietary factors and risk of breast cancer: combined analysis of 12 case control studies. J Natl Cancer Inst 1990; 82: 561–9.

15 Hunter DJ, Spiegelman D, Adami HO, et al. Cohort studies of fat intake and the risk of breast cancer—a pooled analysis. N Engl J Med 1996; 334: 356–61.

16 Trichopoulou A, Katsouyanni K, Stuver S, et al. Consumption of olive oil and specific food groups in relation to breast cancer risk in Greece. J Natl Cancer Inst 1995; 87: 110–16.

17 La Vecchia C, Negri E, Franceschi S, Decarli A, Giacosa A, Lipworth LL. Olive oil, dietary fats and the risk of breast cancer. Cancer Causes Control 1995; 6: 545–50.

18 Wolk A, Bergstrom R, Hunter D, Willett W, et al. A prospective study of association of monounsaturated fat and other types of fat with risk of breast cancer. Arch Intern Med 1998; 158: 41–5.

19 Garland M, Willett WC, Manson JE, Hunter DJ. Antioxidant micronutrients and breast cancer. J Am Coll Nutr 1993; 12: 400–11.

20 Hunter DJ, Manson JE, Colditz GA, et al. A prospective study of the intake of vitamins C, E and A and the risk of breast cancer. N Engl J Med 1993; 329: 234–40.

21 Kushi LH, Fee RM, Sellers TA, Zheng W, Folsom AR. Intake of Vitamins A, C and E and postmenopausal breast cancer. The Iowa Woman's Health Study. Am J Epidemiol 1996; 144: 165–74.

22 Colston KW, Berger U, Coombs RC. Possible role for vitamin D in controlling breast cancer proliferation. Lancet 1989; 1: 188–91.

23 Fraumeni JF, Lloyd JW, Smith EM, et al. Cancer mortality among nuns: role of marital status in etiology of neoplastic disease in women. J Natl Cancer Inst 1969; 42: 455–68.

24 Cole P, MacMahon B. Oestrogen fractions during early reproductive life in the aetiology of breast cancer. Lancet 1969; 1: 604–6.

25 Kelsey JL, Gammon MD, John EM. Reproductive risk factors and breast cancer. Epidemiol Rev 1993; 15: 36–47.

26 Rosner B, Colditz GA, Willett WC. Reproductive risk factors in a prospective study of breast cancer: The Nurses Health Study. Am J Epidemiol 1994; 139: 767–70.

27 London SJ, Colditz GA, Stampfer MJ, et al. Lactation and risk of breast cancer in a cohort of US women. Am J Epidemiol 1990; 132: 17–26.

28 Michels KB, Willett WC, Rosner BA, et al. Prospective assessment of

breast feeding and breast cancer incidence among 89,887 women. Lancet 1996; 347: 431–6.

29 Brinton LA, Potischman NA, Swanson CA, et al. Breast feeding and breast cancer risk. Cancer Causes Control 1995; 6: 199–208.

30 Hsieh C-C, Trichopoulos D, Katsouyanni K, Yuasa S. Age at menarche, age at menopause, height and obesity as risk factors for breast cancer: associations and interactions in an international case-control study. Int J Cancer 1990; 46: 796–800.

31 Meyer F, Moisan J, Marcoux D, Bouchard C. Dietary and physical determinants of menarche. Epidemiology 1990; 1: 377–81.

32 Kvale G, Heuch I. Menstrual factors and breast cancer risk. Cancer 1988; 62: 1625–31.

33 Frisch RE. Weight at menarche: similarity for well nourished and undernourished girls at differing ages, and evidence for historical constancy. Pediatrics 1972; 50: 445–50.

34 Lilienfeld AM. Relationship of cancer of the female breast to artificial menopause and marital status. Cancer 1956; 9: 927–34.

35 Irwin KL, Lee NC, Peterson HB, et al. Hysterectomy, tubal sterilisation and the risk of breast cancer. Am J Epidemiol 1988; 127: 1192–201.

36 Key TJA, Chen J, Wang DY, et al. Sex hormones in women in rural China and Britain. Br J Cancer 1990; 2: 631–6.

37 Bernstein L, Yuan J-M, Ross RK, et al. Serum hormone levels in premenopausal Chinese women in Shanghai and white women in Los Angeles: results from two breast cancer case control studies. Cancer Causes Control 1990; 1: 51–8.

38 Goldin BR, Adlercreutz H, Gorbach SL, et al. The relationship between estrogen levels and diets of Caucasian American and Oriental immigrant women. Am J Clin Nutrition 1986; 44: 945–53.

39 Van Loon AJM, Brug J, Goldbohm RA, van den Brandt PA. Differences in cancer incidence and mortality among socioeconomic groups. Scand J Soc Med 1995; 23: 110–20.

40 Faggiano F, Lemma P, Costa G, Gnavi R, Pagnanelli F. Cancer mortality by educational level in Italy. Cancer Causes Control 1995: 6: 311–20.

41 Wagener DK, Schatzkin A. Temporal trends in the socioeconomic gradient for breast cancer mortality among US women. Am J Public Health 1994; 84: 1003–6.

42 McPherson CP, Swenson KK, Jolitz G, Murray CL. Survival of women ages 40–49 years with breast carcinoma according to method of detection. Cancer 1997; 79: 1923–32.

43 Adami H-O, Malker B, Holmberg L, Persson I, Stone B. The relation between survival and age at diagnosis in breast cancer. New Engl J Med 1986; 315: 559–63.

44 Tabar L, Fagerberg G, Chen H-H, et al. Efficacy of breast cancer screening by age. Cancer 1995; 75: 2507–17.

45 Chu KC, Tarone RE, Kessler LG, et al. Recent trends in US breast cancer incidence, survival and mortality rates. J Natl Cancer Inst 1996; 88: 1571–9.

46 Quinn M, Allen E. Changes in incidence of and mortality from breast cancer in England and Wales since the introduction of screening. UK Association of Cancer Registries. BMJ 1995; 311: 1391–5.

47 Smith CL, Kricker A, Armstrong BK. Breast cancer mortality trends in Australia: 1921 to 1994. MJA 1998; 168: 11–14.

48 Folkman J. Fighting cancer by attacking its blood supply. Scientific American 1996; Sept. 116–19.

49 Time magazine 1998; 20: 20–6.

3 BREASTS AND THEIR MEANING

1 Boyd NF, Lockwood GA, Greenberg CV, Martin LJ, Tritcher DL. Effects of a low-fat high-carbohydrate diet on plasma sex hormones in premenopausal women: results from a randomised controlled trial. Br J Cancer 1997; 76: 127–35.

2 Brunner E, White I, Thorogood M, Bristow A, Curle D, Marmot M. Can dietary interventions change diet and cardiovascular risk factors? A meta-analysis of randomized controlled trials. Am J Public Health 1997; 86: 1415–22.

3 Garner H. The First Stone. Picador, Sydney 1995: 53–4.

4 Bryant H, Brasher P. Breast implants and breast cancer—reanalysis of a linkage study. N Engl J Med 1995; 332: 1535–9.

4 DIET

1 Lea AJ. Dietary factors associated with death-rates from certain neoplasms in man. Lancet 1966; 2: 332–3.

2 Armstrong B, Doll R. Environmental factors and cancer incidence and mortality in different countries, with special reference to dietary practices. Int J Cancer 1975; 15: 617–31.

3 De Waard F, Baanders-van Halewijn EA. A prospective study in general practice of breast cancer risk in postmenopausal women. Int J Cancer 1974; 14: 153–60.

4 Hunter DJ, Willett WC. Diet, body size and breast cancer. Epidemiol Rev 1993; 15: 110–32.

5 Sasaki S, Kesteloot H. Value of Food and Agriculture Organisation data on food balance sheets as a data source for dietary fat intake in epidemiological studies. Am J Clin Nutr 1992; 56: 716–23.

6 Davis WH. The relation of the foreign population to the mortality rates. Bull Am Acad Med 1913; 14: 19–54. Quoted by William Haenszel. Cancer mortality among foreign born in the US. J Natl Cancer Inst 1961; 26: 37–132.

7 Lombard HL, Doering CR. Cancer studies in Massachusetts. Cancer mortality in native groups. J Prev Med 1929; 3: 343–61.

8 Haenszel W. Cancer mortality among the foreign born in the US. J Natl Cancer Inst 1961; 26: 37–132.

9 Haenszel W, Kurihara M. Studies of Japanese migrants. Mortality from cancer and other diseases among Japanese in the US. J Natl Cancer Inst 1968; 40: 43–68.

10 Ziegler RG, Hoover RN, Pike MC, et al. Migration patterns and breast cancer risk in Asian-American women. J Natl Cancer Inst 1993; 83: 1819–27.

11 Shimizu H, Ross RK, Yatani R, Henderson BE, Mack TM. Cancers of the prostate and breast among Japanese and white immigrants in Los Angeles County. Br J Cancer 1991; 63: 963–6.

12 Berrino F, Gatta G. Energy rich diet and breast cancer risk. Letter. Int J Cancer 1989; 44:186–7.

13 Barbone F, Filiberti R, Franceschi S, et al. Socioeconomic status, migration and the risk of breast cancer in Italy. Int J Epidemiol 1996; 25: 479–87.

14 Stanford JL, Herrinton LJ, Schwartz SM, Weiss NS. Breast cancer incidence in Asian migrants to the US and their descendants. Epidemiology 1995; 6: 181–3.

15 Minami Y, Staples MP, Giles GG. The incidence of colon, breast and prostate cancer in Italian migrants to Victoria, Australia. Eur J Cancer 1993; 29A: 1735–40.

16 Hopkins S, Margetts BM, Armstrong BK. Dietary change among Italians and Australians in Perth. Community Health Stud 1980; 4: 67–75.

17 Rutishauser I, Walquist ML. Food intake patterns of Greek migrants to Melbourne in relation to stay. Proc Nutr Soc Aust 1983; 8: 49–55.

18 Cashel K, English R, Bennett S. National dietary survey of adults 1983. Commonwealth of Australia Department of Health 1986, Canberra.

19 Owles EN. A comparative study of nutrient intakes of migrant and Australian children in Western Australia. Med J Aust 1975; 2: 130–3.

20 Hunter DJ, Spiegelman D, Adami H-O, et al. Cohort studies of fat intake and

the risk of breast cancer—a pooled analysis. N Engl J Med 1996; 334: 356–61.

21 Kvale G, Heuch I. Menstrual factors and breast cancer risk. Cancer 1988; 62: 1625–31.

22 Hsieh CC, Trichopoulos D, Katsouyani K, Yuasa S. Age at menarche, age at menopause, height and obesity as risk factors for breast cancer: associations and interactions in an international case-control study. Int J Cancer 1990; 46: 796–800.

23 Rosner B, Colditz GA, Willett WC. Reproductive risk factors in a prospective study of breast cancer: The Nurses Health Study. Am J Epidemiol 1994; 139: 767–70.

24 Frisch RE. Weight at menarche: similarity for well nourished and undernourished girls at differing ages, and evidence for historical constancy. Pediatrics 1972; 50: 445–50.

25 Maclure M, Travis LB, Willett W, MacMahon BE. A prospective cohort study of nutrient intake and age at menarche. Am J Clin Nutr 1991; 54: 649–56.

5 IS THERE PROOF OF THE EFFECTS OF DIET?

1 Singer SR, Grismaijer S. Dressed to kill—the link between breast cancer and bras. Avery, New York, 1995.

2 Hunter DJ, Willett WC. Diet, body size and breast cancer. Epidemiol Rev 1993; 15: 110–32.

3 Hirohata T, Shigematsu T, Nomura AMY, et al. Occurrence of breast cancer in relation to diet and reproductive history: a case-control study in Fukuoka, Japan. Natl Cancer Inst Monogr 1985; 69: 187–90.

4 Wang Q-S, Ross RK, Yu M, Ning J-P, Henderson BE, Kimm HT. A case control study of breast cancer in Tianjin, China. Cancer Epidemiol Biomarkers Prev 1992; 1: 435–9.

5 Kato I, Miura S, Kasumi F, et al. A case-control study of breast cancer among Japanese women: with special reference to family history and reproductive and dietary factors. Breast Cancer Res Treat 1992; 24: 51–9.

6 Yuan J-M, Wang Q-S, Ross RK, Henderson BE, Yu MC. Diet and breast cancer in Shanghai and Tianjin. China. Br J Cancer 1995; 71:1353–8.

7 Yuan J-M, Yu MC, Ross RK, Gao YT, Henderson BE. Risk factors for breast cancer in Chinese women in Shanghai. Cancer Res 1988; 49: 1949–53.

8 Tao SC, Yu MC, Ross RK, Xiu KW. Risk factors for breast cancer in Chinese women in Beijing. Int J Cancer 1988; 42: 495–8.

9 Tannenbaum A. The genesis and growth of tumours II. Effects of calorie restriction per se. Cancer Res 1942; 2: 460–7.

10 Tannenbaum A. The genesis and growth of tumors III. Effects of a high-fat diet. Cancer Res 1942; 2: 468–75.

11 Armstrong B, Doll R. Environmental factors and cancer incidence and mortality in different countries, with special reference to dietary practices. Int J Cancer 1975; 15: 617–31.

12 Howe GR, Hirohata T, Hislop TG, et al. Dietary factors and risk of breast cancer: combined analysis of 12 case control studies. J Natl Cancer Inst 1990; 82: 561–9.

13 Hunter DJ, Spiegelman D, Adami H-O, et al. Cohort studies of fat intake and the risk of breast cancer—a pooled analysis. N Engl J Med 1996; 334: 356–61.

14 Rohan TE, Howe GR, Friedenreich CM, et al. Dietary fiber, vitamins A, C, E and risk of breast cancer: a cohort study. Cancer Causes Control 1993; 4: 29–37.

15 Hunter DJ, Manson J, Colditz GA, et al. A prospective study of the intake of vitamins C, E and A and the risk of breast cancer. New Engl J Med 1993; 329: 234–40.

16 Kushi LH, Fee RM, Sellers TA, Zheng W, Folsom AR. Intake of vitamins A, C and E and postmenopausal breast cancer. Am J Epidemiol 1996; 144: 165–74.

17 Steinmetz KI, Potter JD. Vegetables, fruit and cancer protection: a review. J Am Diet Assoc 1996; 96: 1027–39.

18 Cohen LA, Kendall ME, Zang E, et al. Modulation of N-nitrosomethylurea induced mammary tumor promotion by dietary fiber and fat. J Natl Cancer Inst 1991; 83: 496–501.

19 Willett WC, Hunter DJ, Stampfer MJ, Colditz G, Manson J, Spiegelman D. Dietary fat and fibre in relation to risk of breast cancer. JAMA 1992; 268: 2037–44.

20 Messina M, Barnes S. The role of soy products in reducing risk of cancer. J Natl Cancer Inst 1991; 83: 541–6.

21 Yuan J-M, Wang Q-S, Ross RK, Henderson BE, Yu MC. Diet and breast cancer in Shanghai and Tianjin, China. Br J Cancer 1995; 71: 1353–8.

22 Ingram D, Sanders K, Kolybabba M, Lopez D. Case-control study of phyto-oestrogens and breast cancer. Lancet 1997; 350: 990–4.

23 Lee HP, Gourley L, Duffy SW, et al. Dietary effects on breast cancer risk in Singapore. Lancet 1991; 337: 1197–1200.

23a Hilakivi-Clarke L, Cho E, Clarke R. Maternal genistein exposure mimics the effects of oestrogen on mammary gland development in female mouse offspring. Oncology Reports 1998; 5: 609–16.

24 Martin-Moreno JM, Willett WC, Gorgojo L, et al. Dietary fat, olive oil intake and breast cancer risk. Int J Cancer 1994; 58: 774–80.

25 Landa MC, Frago N, Tres A. Diet and risk of breast cancer in Spain. Eur J Cancer Prev 1994; 3: 313–20.

26 Trichopoulou A, Katsouyanni K, Stuver S, et al. Consumption of olive oil and specific food groups in relation to breast cancer risk in Greece. J Natl Cancer Inst 1995; 87: 110–16.

27 La Vecchia C, Negri E, Franceschi S, et al. Olive oil, dietary fats and the risk of breast cancer. Cancer Causes Control 1995; 6: 545–50.

28 Wolk A, Bergstrom R, Hunter D, et al. A prospective study of association of monounsaturated fat and other types of fat with risk of breast cancer. Arch Int Med 1998; 158: 41–5.

29 Hunter DJ, Morris JS, Stampfer MJ, et al. A prospective study of selenium status and breast cancer risk. JAMA 1990; 264: 1128–31.

30 Hunter DJ, Manson JE, Stampfer MJ, et al. A prospective study of caffeine, coffee, tea and breast cancer (abstract). Am J Epidemiol 1992; 136: 1000–1.

31 Goldbohm RA, Hertog MG, Brandts HA, van Poppel G, van den Brandt PA. Consumption of black tea and cancer risk: a prospective cohort study. J Natl Cancer Inst 1996; 88: 93–100.

32 Zheng W, Doyle TJ, Kushi LH, Sellers TA, Hong CP, Folsom AR. Tea consumption and cancer incidence in a prospective cohort study of postmenopausal women. Amer J Epidemiol 1996; 144: 175–82.

33 Tsubono Y, Takahashi T, Iwase Y, Iitoi Y, Akabane M, Tsugane S. Dietary differences with green tea intake among middle aged Japanese men and women. Preventive Med. 1997; 26: 704–10.

34 Outwater JL, Nicholson A, Barnard N. Dairy products and breast cancer: the IGF-I, estrogen, and bGH hypothesis. Medical Hypotheses 1997; 48: 453–61.

35 Keller HF, Chew BP, Erb RE, Malven PV. Mammary transfer of hormones and constituents into secretions when cows were milked or secretions were sampled prepartum. J Dairy Science 1977; 60: 546–56.

36 Westin JB, Richter E. The Israeli breast-cancer anomaly. Ann NY Acad Sci 1990; 609: 269–79.

37 Tretli S, Gaard M. Lifestyle changes during adolescence and risk of breast cancer: an ecologic study of the effect of World War II in Norway. Cancer Causes Control 1996; 7: 507–12.

38 Kelsey JL, Gammon MD, John EM. Reproductive factors and breast cancer. Epidemiol Rev 1993; 15: 36–47.

39 Li CI, Malone KE, White E, Daling JR. Age when maximum height is reached as a risk factor for breast cancer among US women. Epidemiology 1997; 8: 559–65. 1996; 334: 356–61.

40 Potischman N, Weiss HA, Swanson CA, et al. Diet during adolescence and risk of breast cancer among young women. J Natl Cancer Inst 1998; 90: 226–33.

41 Frankel S, Gunnell DJ, Peters TJ, Maynard M, Davey Smith G. Childhood energy intake and adult mortality from cancer: the Boyd Orr cohort study. BMJ 1998: 316: 499–503.

6 PHYSICAL FACTORS AND SOCIAL CLASS

1 Yong L-C, Brown CC, Schatzkin A, Schairer C. Prospective study of relative weight and risk of breast cancer: the breast cancer detection demonstration project follow up study, 1979 to 1987–1989. Am J Epidemiol 1996; 143: 985–95.

2 Hunter DJ, Willett WC. Diet, body size and breast cancer. Epidemiol Rev 1993; 15: 110–32.

3 Ursin G, Longnecker MP, Haile RW, Greenland S. A meta-analysis of body mass index and risk of premenopausal breast cancer. Epidemiology 1995; 6: 137–41.

4 Yuan JM, Yu MC, Ross RK, Gao YT, Henderson BE. Risk factors for breast cancer in Chinese women in Shanghai. Cancer Res 1988; 49: 1949–53.

5 Kato I, Miura S, Kasumi F, et al. A case-control study of breast cancer among Japanese women: with special reference to family history and reproductive and dietary factors. Breast Cancer Res Treatment 1992; 24: 51–9.

6 Albanes D, Taylor PR. International differences in body height and weight and their relationship to cancer incidence. Nutr Cancer 1990; 14: 69–77.

7 London SJ, Colditz GA, Stampfer MJ, et al. Prospective study of relative weight, height and risk of breast cancer. JAMA 1989; 262: 2853–8.

8 Ziegler RG, Hoover RN, Nomura AMY, et al. Relative weight, weight change, height and breast cancer risk in Asian-American women. J Natl Cancer Inst 1996; 88: 650–60.

9 Palmer JR, Rosenberg L, Harlap S, Strom BL, Warshauer ME, et al. Adult height and risk of breast cancer among US Black women. Am J Epidemiol. 1995; 141: 845–49.

10 Potischman N, Swanson CA, Siiteri P, Hoover RN. Reversal of relation between body mass and endogenous estrogen concentrations with menopausal status. J Natl Cancer Inst 1996; 88: 756–8.

11 Huang Z, Hankinson SE, Colditz GA, et al. Dual effects of weight and weight gain on breast cancer risk. JAMA 1997; 278: 1407–11.

12 Tretli S. Height and weight in relation to breast cancer morbidity and

mortality. A prospective study of 570,000 women in Norway. Int J Cancer 1989; 44: 23–30.

13 Hunter DJ, Willett WC. Diet, body size and breast cancer. Epidemiol Rev 1993; 15: 110–32.

14 Li CI, Malone KE, White E, Daling JR. Age when maximum height is reached as a risk factor for breast cancer among young US women. Epidemiology 1997; 8: 559–65.

15 Beijerinck D, van Noord PAH, Kemmeren JM, Seidell JC. Breast size as a determinant of breast cancer. Int J Obesity 1995; 19: 202–5.

16 Ingleby H, Gershon-Cohen J. Comparative anatomy, pathology and roentgenology of the breast. Philadelphia: University of Philadelphia Press, 1960.

17 Bryant H, Brasher P. Breast implants and breast cancer—reanalysis of a linkage study. N Engl J Med 1995; 332: 1535–9.

18 Deapen DM, Brody GS. Augmentation mammaplasty and breast cancer: a 5 year update of the Los Angeles study. Plst Reconstr Surg 1992; 89: 660–5.

19 Sanchez-Guerrero J, Colditz GA, Karlson EW, Hunter DJ, Speizer FE, Liang MH. Silicon breast implants and the risk of connective tissue disease and symptoms. N Engl J Med 1995; 332: 1666–70.

20 Nyren O, Yin L, Josefsson S, et al. Risk of connective tissue disease and related disorder among women with breast implants: a nationwide retrospective cohort study in Sweden. BMJ 1998; 316: 417–22.

21 Brinton LA, Brown SL. Breast implants and cancer. J Natl Cancer Inst 1998; 89; 1341–9.

22 Lawson JS, Black D. Socioeconomic status: the prime indicator of premature death in Australia. J Biosoc Sci 1993; 25: 539–52.

23 Tao S-C, Yu MC, Ross RK, Xiu K-W. Risk factors for breast cancer in Chinese women of Beijing. Int J Cancer 1988; 42: 495–8.

24 Van Loon AJM, Brug J, Goldbohm RA, van den Brandt P. Differences in cancer incidence and mortality among socioeconomic groups. Scand J Soc Med 1995; 23: 110–20.

25 Wagener DK, Schatzkin A. Temporal trends in the socioeconomic gradient for breast cancer mortality among US women. Am J Public Health 1994; 84: 1003–6.

26 Patrick PR. Heights and weights of Queensland children, with particular reference to the tropics: a report of an anthropometric survey by Queensland school health services. Med J Aust 1951; 2: 324–31.

27 May GMS, O'Hara VM, Dugdale AE. Patterns of growth in Queensland

schoolchildren, 1911 to 1976. Med J Aust 1979; 2: 610–14.

28 Cahn A, Hepburn R. A comparison of diets of two groups of school children. Med J Aust 1960; 2: 334–5.

29 McNaughton JW, Cahn AJ. A study of the food intake and activity of a group of urban adolescents. Br J Nutr 1970; 24: 331 –44.

30 Li CI, Malone KE, White E, Daling JR. Age when maximum height is reached as a risk factor for breast cancer among US women. Epidemiology 1997; 8 :559–65.

31 Thune I, Brenn T, Lund E, Gaard M. Physical activity and the risk of breast cancer. N Eng J Med 1997; 336: 1269–75.

32 Coogan PF, Newcomb PA, Clapp RW, Trentham-Dietz A, Baron JA, Longnecker MP. Physical activity in usual occupation and risk of breast cancer (United States). Cancer Causes Control 1997; 8: 626–31.

33 Chen CL, White E, Malone KE, Daling JR. Leisure-time activity in relation to breast cancer among young women (Washington, United States). Cancer Causes Control 1997; 8: 77–84.

7 REPRODUCTIVE FACTORS

1 Kelsey JL, Gammon MD, John EM. Reproductive risk factors and breast cancer. Epidemiol Rev 1993; 15: 36–47.

2 Michels-Blanck H, Byers T, Mokdad AH, Will JC, Calle EE. Menstrual patterns and breast cancer mortality in a large US corhort. Epidemiology 1996; 7: 543–6.

3 Brinton LA, Schairer C, Hoover RN, et al. Menstrual factors and risk of breast cancer. Cancer Invest 1988; 6: 245–54.

4 Irwin KL, Lee NC, Peterson HB, et al. Hysterectomy, tubal sterilisation, and risk of breast cancer. Am J Epidemiol 1988; 127: 1192–1201.

5 Schneider R, Dorn CR, Taylor DON. Factors influencing canine mammary cancer development and postsurgical survival. J Natl Cancer Inst 1969; 43; 1249–66.

6 Apter D, Vikho R. Early menarche, a risk factor for breast cancer, indicates early onset of ovulatory cycles. J Clin Endocrinol Metab 1983; 57: 82–6.

7 Parazzini F, La Vecchia CL, Negri E, Franceschi S, Tozzi L. Lifelong menstrual pattern and risk of breast cancer. Oncology 1993; 50: 222–5.

8 MacMahon B, Cole P, Brown J. Etiology of breast cancer: a review. J Natl Cancer Inst 1973; 50: 21–42.

9 Rosner B, Colditz GA, Willett WC. Reproductive risk factors in a prospective

study of breast cancer: the Nurses Health Study. Am J Epidemiol 1994; 139: 819–35.

10 Cole P, MacMahon B. Oestrogen fractions during early reproductive life in the aetiology of breast cancer. Lancet 1969; 1: 604–6.

11 Russo J, Tay LK, Russo IH. Differentiation of the mammary gland and susceptibility to carcinogenesis. Breast Cancer Research Treatment 1982; 2: 5–73.

12 Michels KB, Willett WC, Rosner BA, et al. Prospective assessment of breastfeeding and breast cancer incidence among 89,887 women. Lancet 1996; 347: 431–6.

13 Yuan JM, Yu MC, Ross RK, Gao YT, Henderson BE. Risk factors for breast cancer in Chinese women in Shanghai. Cancer Res 1988; 49: 1949–53.

14 Tao SC, Yu MC, Ross RK, Xiu KW. Risk factors for breast cancer in Chinese women in Beijing. Int J Cancer 1988; 42: 495–8.

15 Bucalossi P, Veronisi U. Some observations on cancer of the breast in mothers and daughters. Br J Cancer 1957; 11: 337–47.

15a Titus-Ernstoff L, Elan KM, Newcomb P, et al. Exposure to breast milk in infancy and adult breast cancer risk. J Natl Cancer Inst 1998; 90: 921–4.

16 Freudenheim JL, Marshall JR, Graham S, et al. Exposure to breastmilk in infancy and the risk of breast cancer. Epidemiology 1994; 5: 324–31.

17 Brind J, Chinchilli VM, Severs WB, Summy-Long J. Induced abortion as an independent risk factor for breast cancer: a comprehensive review and meta-analysis. J Epidemiol Community Health 1996; 50: 481–96.

18 Melbye M, Wohlfahrt J, Olsen JH, et al. Induced abortion and the risk of breast cancer. N Engl J Med 1997; 336; 81–5.

19 Fraumeni JF, Lloyd JW, Smith EM, Wagoner JK. Cancer mortality among nuns: role of marital status in etiology of neoplastic disease in women. J Natl Cancer Inst 1969; 42: 455–68.

20 Frisch R, Revelle R. Variation in body weights and the age of the adolescent growth spurt among Latin American and Asian populations, in relation to calorie supplies. Human Biol 1969; 41: 185.

21 Hill P, Wynder EL, Garbaczewski L, et al. Diet and menarche in different ethnic groups. Europ J Cancer 1980; 16: 519–25.

22 Burrell RJW, Healy MJR, Tanner JM. Age of menarche in South African Bantu schoolgirls living in the Transkei reserve. Human Biol 1961; 33: 250.

23 Kvale G, Heuch I. Menstrual factors and breast cancer risk. Cancer 1988; 62: 1625–31.

24 Key TJA, Chen J, Wang DY, Pike MC, Boreham J. Sex hormones in women

in rural China and in Britain. Br J Cancer 1990; 62: 631–6.

25 Dann TC, Roberts DF. Menarcheal age in University of Warwick young women. J Biosoc Sci 1993; 25: 531–8.

26 Crisp AH, Stonehill E. Relation between aspects of nutritional disturbance and menstrual activity in primary anorexia nervosa. BMJ 1971; 2: 149–51.

27 Frisch RE. Weight at menarche: similarity for well nourished and undernourished girls at differing ages, and evidence for historical constancy. Pediatrics 1972; 50: 445–50.

28 Frisch RE, Wyshak G, Vincent L. Delayed menarche and amenorrhoea of ballet dancers. New Eng J Med 1980; 303: 17–19.

29 Frisch RE, Gotz-Welbergen AV, McArthur JW, et al. Delayed menarche and amenorrhoea of college athletes in relation to age of onset of training. JAMA 1981; 246: 1559–63.

30 Thune I, Brenn T, Lund E, Gaard M. Physical activity and the risk of breast cancer. N Eng J Med 1997; 336: 1269–75.

31 Merzenich H, Boeing H, Wahrendorf J. Dietary fat and sports activity as determinants for age of menarche. Am J Epidemiol 1993; 138: 217–24.

32 Kissinger DG, Sanchez A. The association of dietary factors with the age of menarche. Nutrition Research 1987; 7: 471–9.

33 Maclure M, Travis LB, Willett W, MacMahon B. A prospective cohort study of nutrient intake and age at menarche. Am J Clin Nutr 1991; 54: 649–56.

34 Meyer F, Moisan J, Marcoux D, Bouchard C. Dietary and physical determinants of menarche. Epidemiology 1990; 1: 377–81.

35 MacMahon B, Trichopoulos D, Brown J, et al. Age at menarche, probability of ovulation and breast cancer risk. Int J Cancer 1982; 29: 13–16.

36 Apter D, Vihko R. Early menarche, a risk factor for breast cancer, indicates early onset of ovulatory cycles. J Clin Endocrinol Metab 1983; 57: 82–6.

37 Michels-Blanck H, Byers T, Mokdad AH, Will JC, Calle EE. Menstrual patterns and breast cancer mortality in a large US cohort. Epidemiology 1996; 7: 543–6.

38 Parazzini F, La Vecchia CL, Negri E, Franceschi S, Tozzi L. Lifelong menstrual pattern and risk of breast cancer. Oncology 1993; 50: 222–5.

39 Soini I. Risk factors of breast cancer in Finland. Int J Epidemiol 1977; 6: 365–73.

40 Collaborative group on hormonal factors in breast cancer. Lancet 1996; 347: 1713–27.

41 Hankinson SE, Colditz GA, Manson JE, et al. A prospective study of oral contraceptive use and risk of breast cancer (Nurses Health Study, US). Cancer Causes and Control 1997; 8: 65–72.

42 Schurman AG, van den Brandt PA, Goldbohm RA. Exogenous hormone use and the risk of postmenopausal breast cancer: results from the Netherlands Cohort Study. Cancer Causes Control 1995; 6: 416–24.

43 Grodstein F, Stampfer MJ, Colditz GA, et al. Postmenopausal hormone therapy and mortality. N Engl J Med 1997; 336: 1769–75.

44 Beral V, Banks E, Reeves G, Wallis M. Hormone replacement therapy and high incidence of breast cancer between mammographic screens (letter). Lancet 1997; 349: 1103–4.

8 FROM ATOM BOMBS TO ALCOHOL

1 McGregor DH, Land CE, Choi K, et al. Breast cancer incidence among atomic bomb survivors, Hiroshima and Nagasaki, 1950–69. J Natl Cancer Inst 1977; 59: 799–811.

2 Hildreth NG, Shore RE, Dvoretsky PM. The risk of breast cancer after irradiation of the thymus in infancy. N Engl J Med 1989; 321: 1281–4.

3 Miller AB, Howe GR, Sherman GJ, Lindsay JP, Yaffe MJ, Dinner PJ. Mortality from breast cancer after irradiation during fluoroscopic examinations in patients being treated for tuberculosis. N Engl J Med 1989; 321: 1285–9.

4 Land CE, Boice JD, Shore RE, Norman JE, Tokunaga M. Breast cancer risk from low-dose exposures to ionising radiation: results of parallel analysis of three exposed populations of women. J Natl Cancer Inst 1980; 65: 353–68.

5 Longnecker MP, Newcomb PA, Mittendorf R, et al. Risk of breast cancer in relation to lifetime alcohol consumption. J Natl Cancer Inst 1995; 87: 923–9.

6 Longnecker MP. Alcoholic beverage consumption in relation to risk of breast cancer: meta-analysis and review. Cancer Causes Control 1994; 5: 73–82.

7 Swanson CA, Coates RJ, et al. Alcohol consumption and breast cancer risk among women under age 45 years. Epidemiology 1997; 8: 231–7.

8 Williams RR, Horm JW. Association of cancer sites with tobacco and alcohol consumption and socioeconomic status of patients: interview study from the Third National Cancer Survey. J Natl Cancer Inst 1977; 58: 525–47.

9 Smith-Warner SA, Spiegelman D, Yaun S-S, et al. Alcohol and breast cancer in women. JAMA 1998; 278: 535–40.

10 Reichman ME, Judd JT, Longcope C, et al. Effects of alcohol consumption on plasma and urinary hormone concentrations in premenopausal women. J Natl Cancer Inst 1993; 85: 722–7.

11 Thun MJ, Peto R, Lopez AD, et al. Alcohol consumption and mortality among middle-aged and elderly US adults. N Eng J Med 1997; 337: 1705–14.

12 Fuchs CS, Stampfer MJ, Colditz GA, et al. Alcohol consumption and mortality among women. N Engl J Med 1995; 332: 1245–50.

9 WORLD WAR II AND LEFTIST TENDENCIES

 1 Tretli S. Height and weight in relation to breast cancer morbidity and mortality. A prospective study of 570,000 women in Norway. Int J Cancer 1989; 45: 23–30.

 2 Vatten LJ, Kvinnsland S. Body height and risk of breast cancer. A prospective study of 23,831 Norwegian women. Br J Cancer 1990; 61: 881–5.

 3 Tretli S, Gaard M. Lifestyle changes during adolescence and risk of breast cancer: an ecological study of the effect of the Second World War in Norway. Cancer Causes Control 1996; 7: 507–12.

 4 Hansen OG. Food conditions in Norway during the war 1939–45. Proc Nutr Soc 1947; 5: 263–7.

 5 Strom A. Examination into the diet of Norwegian families during the war years 1942–45. Acta Med Scan 1948; Supp. 114: 1–47.

 6 Bruntland GH, Liestol K, Walloe L. Height, weight and menarcheal age of Oslo schoolchildren during the last 60 years. Ann Human Biol 1980; 7: 307–22.

 7 World Health Statistics Annuals 1987–1994. WHO Geneva.

 8 Jansen BCP. Nutritional research in Holland during the war. Proc Nutr Soc 1947; 5: 305–11.

 9 Marrack JR. Investigations of human nutrition in the United Kingdom during the war. Proc Nutr Soc 1947; 5: 213–41.

10 Van Noord PAH, Kaaks R. The effect of wartime conditions and the 1944–45 'Dutch famine' on recalled menarcheal age in participants of the DOM breast cancer screening project. Ann Human Biol 1991; 18: 57–70.

11 Lumey LH, Stam GA, Ravelli AC, Stein ZA. Birth weight, birth cohort and adult weight among women born during the Dutch famine of 1944–45. Am J Epidemiol 1992; 136: 951 (abstract).

12 Skjaerven R, Wilcox AJ, Oyen N, Magnus P. Mothers' birthweight and survival of their offspring: population based study. BMJ 1997; 314:1376–80.

13 Jones AP, Friedman MI. Obesity and adipocyte abnormalities in offspring of rats undernourished during pregnancy. Science 1982; 219: 1093–4.

14 Weiss HA, Devesa SS, Brinton LA. Laterality of breast cancer in the United States. Cancer Causes Control 1996; 7: 539–43.

15 Brisson J, Verreault R, Morrison AS, Tennina S, Meyer F. Diet, mammographic features of breast tissue, and breast cancer risk. Am J Epidemiol 1989; 130: 14–24.

16 Ekbom A, Adami H-O, Trichopoulos D, Lambe M, Hsieh C-C, Ponten J. Epidemiologic correlates of breast cancer laterality (Sweden). Cancer Causes Control 1994; 5: 510–16.

17 Hsieh C-C, Trichopoulos D. Breast size, handedness and breast cancer risk. Eur J Cancer 1991; 27: 131–5.

18 Petridou E, Flytzani V, Youroukos S, et al. Birth weight and handedness in boys and girls. Human Biology 1994; 66: 1093–101.

10 OLD AND NEW IDEAS

1 Howe GR, Hirohata T, Hislop TG, et al. Dietary factors and risk of breast cancer: combined analysis of 12 case control studies. J Natl Cancer Inst 1990; 82: 561–9.

2 Hunter DJ, Spiegelman D, Adami H-O, et al. Cohort studies of fat intake and the risk of breast cancer—a pooled analysis. N Engl J Med 1996; 334: 356–61.

3 Garland M, Morris JS, Colditz GA, et al. Toenail trace element levels and breast cancer: a prospective study. Am J Epidemiol 1996; 144: 653–60.

4 Palmer JR, Rosenberg L. Cigarette smoking and the risk of breast cancer. Epidemiol Rev 1993; 15: 145–56.

5 Benicke K, Conrad C, Sabroe S, Sorensen HT. Cigarette smoking and breast cancer. BMJ 1995; 310: 1431–3.

6 Baron JA, La Vecchia C, Levi F. The antiestrogenic effect of cigarette smoking in women. Am J Obstet Gynecol 1990; 162: 502–14.

7 Prescott E, Hippe M, Schnohr P, Hein HO, Vestbo J. Smoking and risk of myocardial infarction in women and men: longitudinal population study. BMJ 1998; 316: 1043–7.

8 De Waard F, Trichopoulos D. A unifying concept of the aetiology of breast cancer. Int J Cancer 1988; 41: 666–9.

9 Berrino F, Gatta G. Energy rich diet and breast cancer risk. Letter. Int J Cancer 1989; 44: 186–7.

10 Barbone F, Filiberti R, Franceschi S, et al. Socioeconomic status, migration and the risk of breast cancer in Italy. Int J Epidemiol 1996; 25: 479–87.

11 Trichopoulos D. Hypothesis: does breast cancer originate in utero? Lancet 1990; 335: 939–90.

12 Petridou E, Panagiotopoupou K, Katsouyanni K, Spanos E, Trichopoulos D. Tobacco smoking, pregnancy estrogens and birth weight. Epidemiology 1990; 1: 247–50.

13 Ekbom A, Trichopoulos D, Adami H-O, Hsieh CC, Lan SJ. Evidence of perinatal influences on breast cancer risk. Lancet 1992; 340: 1015–18.

14 Sandson TA, Wen PY, Lemay M. Reversed cerebral asymmetry in women with breast cancer. Lancet 1992; 339: 523–4.

15 Michels KB, Trichopoulos D, Robins JM, et al. Birthweight as a risk factor for breast cancer. Lancet 1996; 348: 1542–6.

16 Sanderson M, Williams MA, Malone KE, et al. Perinatal risk factors and risk of breast cancer. Epidemiology 1996; 7: 34–7.

17 Ekbom A, Hsieh C-C, Lipworth L, Adami H-O, Trichopoulos D. Intrauterine environment and breast cancer risk in women: a population based study. J Natl Cancer Inst 1997; 88: 71–76.

18 Swerdlow AJ, De Stavola BL, Swanick MA, Maconochie NES. Risks of breast and testicular cancers in young adult twins in England and Wales: evidence on prenatal and genetic aetiology. Lancet 1997; 350: 1723–8.

19 Osborne RH, De George FV. Cancer and contagious disease in twins. Cancer 1967; 20: 263–70.

20 Anazhagen R, Nathan B, Gusterson BA. Perinatal influences and breast cancer (letter). Lancet 1992; 340: 1477–8.

21 Wang X, Guyer B, Paige DM. Differences in gestational age-specific birthweight among Chinese, Japanese and white Americans. Int J Epidemiol 1994; 23: 119–28.

22 Boeryd B, Hallgren B. The incidence of spontaneous mammary carcinoma in C3H mice is influenced by dietary fat given from weaning and given to the mothers during gestation and lactation. Acta Path Microbiol Immunol Scand Sect A 1986; 94: 237–41.

23 Walker BE. Tumors in female offspring of control and diethylstilboestrol-exposed mice fed high-fat diets. J Natl Cancer Inst 1990; 82: 50–4.

24 Hilakivi-Clarke L, Clarke R, Onojaf I, Raygada M, Cho E, Lippman M. A maternal diet high in n-6 polyunsaturated fats alters mammary gland development, puberty onset and breast cancer risk among female rat offspring. Proc Natl Academy Sciences USA 1997; 94: 9372–7.

25 Ravelli G-P, Stein ZA, Susser MW. Obesity in young men after famine exposure in utero and early infancy. N Eng J Med 1976; 295: 349–53.

26 Van Assche FA. Birthweight as risk factor for breast cancer. Lancet 1997; 349: 502.

27 Berstein LM. Newborn macrosomy and cancer. Advances Cancer Res 1988; 50: 231–78.

28 Wolk A, Bergstrom R, Hunter D, et al. A prospective study of association of monounsaturated fat and other types of fat with risk of breast cancer. Arch Intern Med 1998; 158: 41–5.

29 Bulmer MG. Twinning rate in Europe during the war. BMJ 1959; 1: 29–30.

30 Hankinson SE, Willett WC, Colditz GA, et al. Circulating concentrations of insulin-like growth factor-I and risk of breast cancer. Lancet 1998; 351: 1393–6.

31 Ruggeri B, Klurfeld D, Kritchevsky D, Furlavetto RW. Calorie restriction and 7,12-dimethylbenz(a)anthracene-induced mammary tumor growth in rats: alterations in circulation of insulin, insulin-like growth factors I and II and epidermal growth factor. Cancer Res 1998; 49: 4135–41.

32 Rich-Edwards JW, Stampfer MJ, Manson JE, et al. Birth weight and risk of cardiovascular disease in a cohort of women followed up since 1976. BMJ 1997; 315: 396–400.

33 Sorensen HT, Sabroe S, Olsen J, Rothman KJ, Gillman MW, Fischer P. Birth weight and cognitive function in young adult life: historical cohort study. BMJ 1997; 315: 401–3.

34 Adami HO, Persson I, Ekbom A, Wolk A, Ponten J, Trichopoulos D. The aetiology and pathogenesis of human breast cancer. Mutat Res 1995; 333: 29–35.

35 Haenszel W. Cancer mortality among the foreign born in the United States. J Natl Cancer Inst 1961; 26: 37-132.

36 4. McMichael AJ, Giles GC. Cancer in migrants to Australia: extending the descriptive data. Cancer Research 1988; 48: 751–6.

37 Hopkins S, Margetts BM, Armstrong BK. Dietary change among Italians and Australians in Perth. Community Health Stud 1980; 4: 67-75.

38 Rutishauser I, Walquist ML. Food intake patterns of Greek migrants to Melbourne in relation to stay. Proc Nutr Soc Aust 1983; 8: 49-55.

39 Herbst AL, Ulfelder H, Poskanzer DC. Adenocarcinoma of the vagina. Association of maternal stilbestrol therapy with tumor appearance in young women. N Engl J Med 1971; 284: 878–81.

40 Ross JA, Perentis JP, Robison LL, Davies SM. Big babies and infant leukaemia: a role for insulin-like growth factor-1? Cancer Causes Control 1996; 7: 553–9.

41 Leisenring WM, Breslow NE, Evans IE, Beckwith JB, Coppes MJ, Grundy P. Increased birth weights of National Wilm's Tumor Study patients suggest a growth factor excess. Cancer Res 1994; 54: 4680–3.

42 Skjaerven R, Wilcox AJ, Oyen N, Magnus P. Mothers' birthweight and survival of their offspring: population based study. BMJ; 1997: 314:1376–80.

43 Stein Z, Susser M. The Dutch famine, 1944-1945, and the reproductive process. I. Effects on six indices at birth. Pediat Res 1975; 9: 70–6.

44 Lumey LH, Stam GA, Ravelli ACJ, Santana SM, Stein Z. Birth cohort, birth weight and offspring birthweight of women born during the Dutch famine of

1944-45. Abstract Paediatr Perinat Epidemiol 1993; 7: A3-4.

45 Little RE. Mothers and fathers birth weight as predictors of infant birth weight. Paediatr Perinat Epidemiol 1987; 1: 19-31.

46 Magnus P, Berg K, Bjerkedal T, Lance WE. Parental determinants of birth weight. Paediatr Perinat Epidemiol 1989; 3: 432–47.

11 SO WHAT DO WE KNOW?

1 Cole P, MacMahon B. Oestrogen fractions during early reproductive life in the aetiology of breast cancer. Lancet 1969; 1: 604–6.

2 Hunter DJ, Willett WC. Diet, body size and breast cancer. Epidemiol Rev 1993; 15: 110–32.

3 Adami H-O, Persson I, Ekbom A, Wolk A, Ponten J, Trichopoulos D. The aetiology and pathogenesis of human breast cancer. Mutation Research 1995; 333: 29–35.

4 Goldin BR, Adlercreutz H, Gorbach SL, et al. The relationship between estrogen levels and diets of Caucasian American and Oriental immigrant women. Am J Clin Nutr 1986; 44: 945–53.

5 Key TJA, Chen J, Wang DY, Pike MC, Boreham J. Sex hormones in women in rural China and in Britain. Br J Cancer 1990; 62: 631–6.

6 Bernstein L, Yuan J-M, Ross RR, et al. Serum hormone levels in premenopausal Chinese women in Shanghai and white women in Los Angeles: results from two breast cancer case-control studies. Cancer Causes Control 1990; 1: 51–8.

7 Brind J, Chinchilli VM, Severs WB, Summy-Long J. Induced abortion as an independent risk factor for breast cancer: a comprehensive review and meta-analysis. J Epidemiol Community Health 1996; 50: 481–96.

8 Melbye M, Wohlfahrt J, Olsen JH, et al. Induced abortion and the risk of breast cancer. N Engl J Med 1997; 336: 81–5.

9 Armstrong B, Doll R. Environmental factors and cancer incidence and mortality in different countries, with special reference to dietary practices. Int J Cancer 1975;15: 617–31.

10 World Health Statistics Annual 1995. WHO 1996, Geneva.

11 Food Tables. Food and Agriculture Organisation of the United Nations. Rome 1996.

12 Haenszel W. Cancer mortality among the foreign born in the US. J Natl Cancer Inst 1961; 26: 37–132.

13 Michels KB, Trichopoulos D, Robins JM, et al. Birthweight as a risk factor for breast cancer. Lancet 1996; 348: 1542–6.

14 Hilakivi-Clarke L, Clarke R, Onojaf I, et al. A maternal diet high in n-6 polyunsaturated fats alters mammary gland development, puberty onset and breast cancer risk among female rat offspring. Proc Natl Academy Sciences USA 1997; 94: 9372–7.

15 Huggins C, Grand LC, Brillantes FP. Mammary cancer induced by a single feeding of polynuclear hydrocarbons and its suppression. Nature 1961;189: 204–7.

16 Grubbs CJ, Peckham JC, Cato KD. Mammary carcinogenesis in relation to age at time of N-nitroso-N methyl urea administration. J Natl Cancer Inst 1983; 70: 209–12.

17 Dao TL. Mammary cancer induction by 7,12-Dimethylbenz(a)anthracene: relation to age. Science 1969; 165: 810–11.

18 Ip C, Ip M. Inhibition of mammary tumorigenesis by a reduction of fat intake after carcinogen treatment in young versus adult rats. Cancer Letters 1980; 11: 35–42.

19 Dao T, Chan P. Effect of duration of high fat intake on enhancement of mammary carcinogenesis in rats. J Natl Cancer Inst 1983; 71: 201–5.

20 Shimizu H, Ross RK, Yatani R, Henderson BE, Mack TM. Cancers of the prostate and breast among Japanese and white immigrants in Los Angeles County. Br J Cancer 1991; 63: 963–6.

21 Ziegler RG, Hoover RN, Pike MC, et al. Migration patterns and breast cancer risk in Asian-American women. J Natl Cancer Inst 1993; 83: 1819–27.

22 Barbone F, Filiberti R, Franceschi S, et al. Socioeconomic status, migration and the risk of breast cancer in Italy. Int J Epidemiol 1996; 25: 479–87.

23 Frisch RE. The right weight: body fat, menarche and ovulation. Bailliere's Clin Obstet Gynaecol 1990; 4: 419–39.

24 Maclure M, Travis LB, Willett W, MacMahon B. A prospective cohort study of nutrient intake and age at menarche. Am J Clin Nutr 1991; 54: 649–56.

25 Meyer F, Moisan J, Marcoux D, Bouchard C. Dietary and physical determinants of menarche. Epidemiology 1990; 1: 377–81.

26 Hill P, Wynder EL, Garbaczewski L, et al. Diet and menarche in different ethnic groups. Europ J Cancer 1980; 16: 519–25.

27 Gray GE, Pike MC, Hirayama T, et al. Diet and hormone profiles in teenage girls in four countries at different risk for breast cancer. Prev Med 1982; 11: 108–13.

28 Hoel DG, Wakabayashi T, Pike MC. Secular trends in the distributions of the breast cancer risk factors—menarche, first birth, menopause, and weight—in Hiroshima and Nagasaki, Japan. Am J Epidemiol 1983; 118: 78–89.

29 Frisch RE, McArthur JW. Menstrual cycles: fatness as a determinant of minimum weight for height necessary for their maintenance or onset. Science 1974; 185: 949–51.

30 Li CI, Malone KE, White E, Daling JR. Age when maximum height is reached as a risk factor for breast cancer among US women. Epidemiology 1997; 8: 559 66. 1996; 334: 356–61.

31 McGregor DH, Land CE, Choi K, et al. Breast cancer incidence among atomic bomb survivors, Hiroshima and Nagasaki, 1950–69. J Natl Cancer Inst 1977; 59: 799–811.

32 Land CE, Boice JD, Shore RE, Norman JE, Tokunaga M. Breast cancer risk from low-dose exposures to ionising radiation: results of parallel analysis of three exposed populations of women. J Natl Cancer Inst 1980; 65: 353–68.

33 Irwin KL, Lee NC, Peterson HB, et al. Hysterectomy, tubal sterilisation and the risk of breast cancer. Am J Epidemiol 1988; 127: 1192–201.

34 Schneider R, Dorn CR, Taylor DON. Factors influencing canine mammary cancer development and postsurgical survival. J Natl Cancer Inst 1969; 43; 1249–61.

35 Herbst AL, Ulfelder H, Poskanzer DC. Adenocarcinoma of the vagina. Association of maternal stilbestrol therapy with tumor appearance in young women. N Engl J Med 1971; 284: 878–81.

36 Ross JA, Perentis JP, Robison LL, Davies SM. Big babies and infant leukaemia: a role for insulin-like growth factor-1? Cancer Causes Control 1996; 7: 553–9.

37 Leisenring WM, Breslow NE, Evans IE, Beckwith JB, Coppes MJ, Grundy P. Increased birth weights of National Wilm's Tumor Study patients suggest a growth factor excess. Cancer Res 1994; 54: 4680–3.

38 Welsch CW. Relationship between dietary fat and experimental mammary tumorigenesis: a review and critique. Cancer Research (Suppl) 1992; 52: 2040s–8s.

39 Messina M, Barnes S. The role of soy products in reducing risk of cancer. J Natl Cancer Inst 1991; 83: 541–6.

40 Colston KW, Berger U, Coombs RC. Possible role for vitamin D in controlling breast cancer proliferation. Lancet 1989; 1: 188–91.

41 Garland M, Willett WC, Manson JE, Hunter DJ. Antioxidant micronutrients and breast cancer. J Am Coll Nutr 1993; 12: 400–11.

42 Hunter DJ, Manson JE, Colditz GA, et al. A prospective study of the intake of vitamins C, E and A and the risk of breast cancer. N Engl J Med 1993; 329: 234–40.

12 POSSIBILITIES FOR CONTROL AND PREVENTION

1 Ford LG, Johnson KA. Tamoxifen Breast Cancer Prevention Trial—an update. Progress Clinical Biol Research 1997; 396: 271–82.

2 Early Breast Cancer Trialists Collaborative Group. Tamoxifen for early breast cancer: an overview of randomised trials. Lancet 1998; 351: 1451–67.

3 Wang TT, Phang JM. Effect of N-(4 hydroxyphenyl) retinamide on apoptosis in human breast cells. Cancer Letters 1996; 107: 65–71.

4 Boyd NF, Lockwood GA, Greenberg CV, Martin LJ, Tritcher DL. Effects of a low-fat high-carbohydrate diet on plasma sex hormones in premenopausal women: results from a randomised controlled trial. Br J Cancer 1997; 76: 127–35.

5 Brunner E, White I, Thorogood M, Bristow A, Curle D, Marmot M. Can dietary interventions change diet and cardiovascular risk factors? A meta-analysis of randomized controlled trials. Am J Public Health 1997; 86: 1415–22.

6 Kissinger DG, Sanchez A. The association of dietary factors with the age of menarche. Nutrition Research 1987; 7: 471–9.

13 WHAT CAN I DO NOW?

1 Australian National Breast Cancer Centre. Breast changes. What you need to know. Sydney 1997.

2 NSW Cancer Council. Understanding breast cancer. Sydney 1991.

index

abortion, 97–8, 160, 169–70

Adami, Hans-Olaf, 139, 140, 142, 143, 156–7, 159

adrenal glands, 23

AIDS virus, 131–2

alcohol consumption, 53, 54, 82, 114–17, 167, 170, 177

anorexia nervosa, 101, 165, 180

anti-angiogenesis, 36, 197

anti-oestrogens, 63, 135, 171–2

antioxidants, 60, 61, 66, 168, 197

Apter, Dan, 104

Armstrong, Bruce, 43–5, 58

Beatson, GT, 22

Beijerinck, David, 78

Berrino, Franco, 136

Berstein, Lev, 147

biopsy, 6, 197
  core aspiration, 193
  incisional, 6–7, 193
  needle, 193

birth, age at first full-term, 89, 92–4, 100, 155, 157, 169, 178

birth weight, 2, 124–5, 142, 143, 151, 176
  and cardiovascular disease, 150
  and hand-use, 126

births, number of, 95

Boyd Orr, Lord, 70

bra theory, 55–6

Bradford Hill, A, 162
  biological gradient, 163, 166
  evaluation of evidence, 162–8

brain symmetry, 143

breast augmentation, 78–9

breast cancer, 17-19, 20, 21, 24, 38, 194–5, 197
  accepted risk factors, 33
  age distribution, 22-4
  environmental factors, 27–8, 50–1, 157
  familial, 8, 24–5, 27, 94, 167
  investigation, 190–3
  late stage promotion, 75, 200
  more common in left breast, 125–6
  multi-generational effect, 149, 150–2, 165–6
  spread, 12, 13, 15–16
  statistics, 15, 21, 23, 43, 46
  survival rates, 16, 34–5, 135
  well established facts, 153–4

breast cancer prevention, xiii–xiv, 16, 33, 116, 134, 148, 171, 183, 185
  main principles, 175–82
  older women, 181–2

breast examination, 190–2

breast lumps *see* lump, in breast

breastfeeding, 3, 5, 30, 95–6, 161, 169, 178
  breast milk, 96–7, 169

breasts, 38
  and advertising, 39
  anatomy, 19–22
  in art, 40-2
  development, 39–40
  self-examination, xiii, 18, 33, 34, 186–8
  size, 77–8, 126